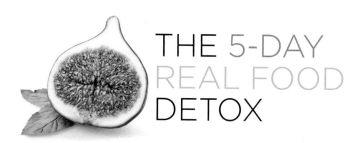

THE 5-DAY
REAL FOOD
DETOX

THE 5-DAY
REAL FOOD
DETOX

NIKKI SHARP

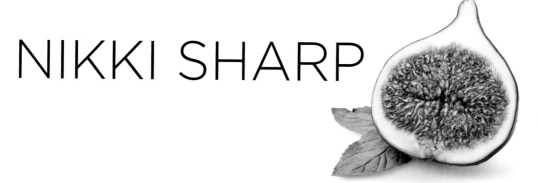

BALLANTINE BOOKS ☖ NEW YORK

No book can replace the diagnostic expertise and medical advice of a trusted physician. Please be certain to consult with your doctor before making any decisions that affect your health or extreme changes in your diet, particularly if you suffer from any medical condition or have any symptom that may require treatment.

As of the time of initial publication, the URLs displayed in this book link or refer to existing websites on the Internet. Penguin Random House LLC is not responsible for, and should not be deemed to endorse or recommend, any website other than its own or any content available on the Internet (including without limitation at any website, blog page, information page) that is not created by Penguin Random House.

A Ballantine Books Trade Paperback Original

Copyright © 2016 by Nikki Sharp

All rights reserved.

Published in the United States by Ballantine Books, an imprint of Random House, a division of Penguin Random House LLC, New York.

BALLANTINE and the HOUSE colophon are registered trademarks of Penguin Random House LLC.

LIBRARY OF CONGRESS CATALOGING-IN-PUBLICATION DATA
Names: Sharp, Nikki.
Title: The 5-day real food detox / Nikki Sharp.
Other titles: Five day real food detox
Description: New York : Ballantine Books, [2016] | Includes bibliographical references and index.
Identifiers: LCCN 2015049293 (print) | LCCN 2015050076 (ebook) | ISBN 9781101886922 (pbk. : alk. paper) | ISBN 9781101886939 (ebook)
Subjects: LCSH: Detoxification (Health) | Diet. | Health.
Classification: LCC RA784.5 .S525 2016 (print) | LCC RA784.5 (ebook) | DDC 613.2—dc23
LC record available at http://lccn.loc.gov/2015049293

Printed in the United States of America on acid-free paper

randomhousebooks.com

9 8 7 6 5 4 3 2 1

Book design by Liz Cosgrove

To everyone who has written me an email, commented on social media, or asked for my advice, my friends and family who look to me for help, and those of you who share your stories with me—this book is dedicated to you. You allow me to share my passion and give me constant inspiration to keep persevering to make the world a better place. Thank you from the bottom of my heart for helping me figure out what I am on this planet to do.

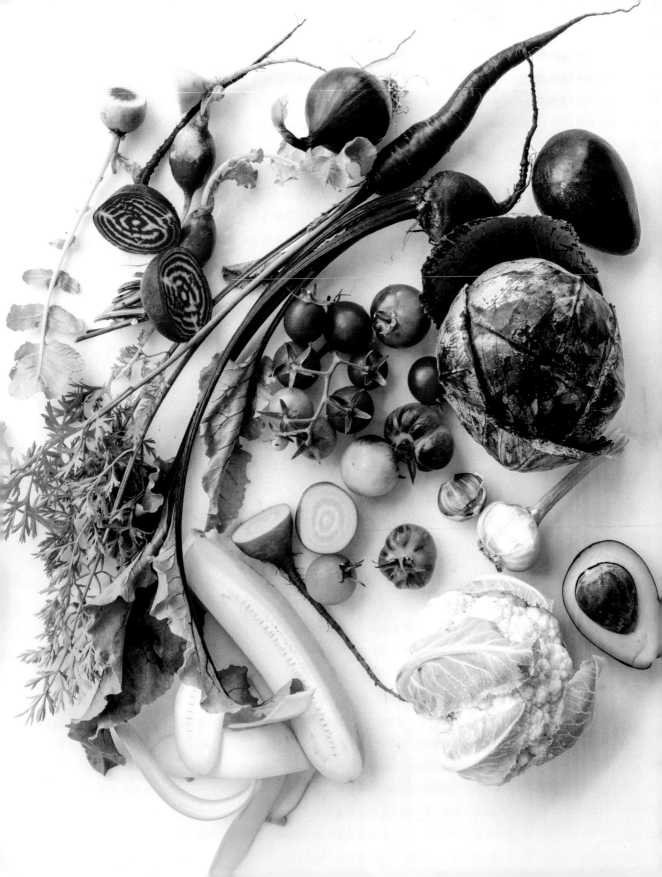

CONTENTS

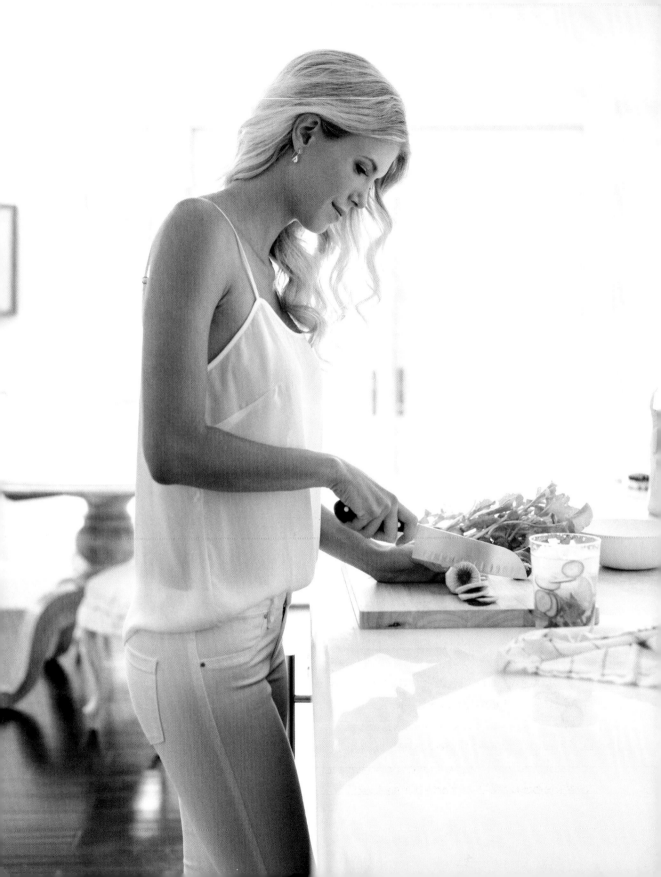

INTRODUCTION
MY STORY

My name is Nikki Sharp, and I'm a model on a mission: to help you detox safely and sanely. And do it in a very unique way—by eating delicious, natural foods that help you shed pounds quickly and radically improve your health and your life. So, welcome! I'm going to show you how to do my *5-Day Real Food Detox,* a fun, healthy process that will change the way you look and feel in five short days. I promise!

I know what you're thinking. Is this some sort of starvation diet only a model would do? Am I going to subsist on celery sticks, cigarettes, and endless cups of coffee? Or is this just another one of those juice-only, smoothie-only detoxes that will leave me feeling unhappy and craving real, chewable food?

No! That's not what I'm about, and it's not what I think life is about. Life is about experiencing health, joy, happiness, and energy—and loving yourself. And one of the most important ways to have that kind of life is to enjoy beautiful, nutrient-dense food.

On my detox, you'll learn simple principles of clean eating. You'll eat real foods that are as close to their natural state as possible—foods that burn body fat, remove toxins, reduce bloating, and clear up nagging conditions such as acne, fatigue, and constipation. You'll start to completely turn your health around. You'll look great, feel great, and have more energy, whether you're 22 or 62. And all of this in just five days.

A MODEL DIET

I developed this cleanse after many years on the modeling circuit, where I ate low-nutrition crap or nothing at all. My typical diet ranged from too many coffees and diet sodas to packs of salted peanuts and fruit yogurts with far too few calories to nightly "snacks" of cupcakes, cookies, pizza, and blocks of cheese with far too many calories. Not exactly good nutrition, and it took a toll on my body and mind: I became very sick and unhappy. On the outside, I seemed to have it all: money, fame, beauty, and a glamorous lifestyle. But on the inside, I was a physical and emotional mess. It would take me many years to "clean up" that mess.

I grew up in Boulder, Colorado. I'm the daughter of an Olympic-cyclist, sports-model mother; a rock-climbing father; and a body-building stepfather. My mother and father are English, originally from London, but moved years ago to the beautiful Rocky Mountains. Boulder, of course, is wonderful for skiing, hiking, cycling, eating great locally sourced food, and living a healthy lifestyle. I wouldn't change that upbringing for the world.

But did I appreciate it back then? Not one bit.

As a kid, I was a typical picky eater. My mother cooked for me every single night—dishes like homemade pasta with fresh tomato sauce and grilled salmon with vegetables—yet I refused to eat her nutritious meals, subsisting instead on chocolatey cereals, low-fat milk, boxed mac and cheese, artichokes with full-fat mayonnaise dip, and Lunchables. Empty nutrition, for sure, and it began to hurt me from a very young age. When I was seven, I was rushed to the emergency room for severe acid reflux. In retrospect, I'm convinced that my poor diet caused it. But back then, no doctor would ever make the connection, especially for someone that young. The link between poor nutrition and illness wasn't as clear as it is now. So like most sick little kids, I was given a stuffed animal and very strong medicine, and sent on my way. It was the typical Band-Aid approach to medical care, which never works. My acid reflux got so bad that by age twelve, I was put on the highest dose of prescription heartburn drugs, and I took them four times a day.

When I was eleven, I got serious acne, which plagued me off and on for the next fifteen years. It wasn't only on my face but all over my back, too. I tried everything to clear it up, from products hyped by beautiful models and actresses on TV to antibiotics and prescription skin gels. I finally resorted to taking Accutane, a very risky and potentially dangerous anti-acne drug, three times a day. Nothing worked. I honestly thought I was just unlucky and would be cursed with acne, terrible stomachaches, and later headaches for the rest of my life. It never occurred to me to ask *why* these things were happening.

My blemish-ridden face and other health problems, however, did not destroy my dream of becoming a model—a dream that took hold very early in my life. For one thing, I was always very tall and naturally thin, exactly the body type for modeling. My mother's career as a sports model influenced me greatly. But more than anything, I was motivated by the glossy magazine spreads of Cindy Crawford, Kate Moss, and Naomi Campbell, and I plastered their pictures all over my bedroom wall. I'd stare at those pictures and tell myself that one day I'd become a model too.

And so, from a very young age, I fantasized about the exciting world of runways, flashing cameras, and designer clothes. I've always been really driven, so at age fifteen, with the encouragement of my family and friends, I went for it. Happily, I learned that multiple layers of makeup could hide my skin problems to an extent during castings. And that with the click of a mouse, Photoshop could erase even my slightest imperfections. Technology could create beautiful photos that showed a girl with crazy amounts of confidence, clear skin, and an even thinner body than I already had.

I began with shoots for local magazines and catalogs, and that work got the attention of modeling agencies in Los Angeles. So at age nineteen, I packed up and headed on my own to California.

One of the (many) pressures of modeling is that you never know how long your career will last. Fashion models typically top out at age twenty-one, so you know the day will come when you stop getting work. I wanted to be prepared to do something else, so I graduated from high school and enrolled in college, majoring in communications and journalism, while modeling. I sailed through my studies fast and furiously, attending three universities in four years and earning my bachelor of arts at age twenty.

I started college at the University of Colorado in Boulder, my hometown, but transferred to the University of Northern Colorado to be with friends. In my junior year, I did an exchange program out to Los Angeles so that I could immerse myself in the world of modeling and acting and begin living the Hollywood dream. Afterward, I headed back to Colorado to graduate from UNC with honors. The whole experience was hectic but taught me a lot, since I was going to school full-time, transferring schools like it was my job, making new friends at each place, modeling on the side, and always working to pay my tuition.

During this period of my life, I figured out that controlling what I ate made me feel in control of my life. My basic menu each day consisted of iceberg lettuce salads, an egg or two, pepperoni slices, cheesy croutons, milk, a few slices of bright orange American cheese, and lots of cups of instant coffee. I probably went through ten packets of artificial sweetener in a day. I was still taking antacids and popping ibuprofen like candy for headaches—and wondering why I felt lousy. I was clueless about proper nutrition or how to feed my body. I just thought: *Eat less, do loads of cardio, and I'll be fine.*

THE WORLD COMES CALLING

My agent always wanted me to model overseas, but I kept telling her that I needed to finish college first. A month after graduation, I was on a plane to Asia. Once you're accepted in an agency in another country, you're given the title "international model," which sounds more desirable to casting directors because a foreign face can give a brand's ad campaign or runway show a fresh, new look. I was even given different names in different countries. For example, while I lived in China, I was called Rose, which is my middle name, to show that I was European. While I modeled in Australia, the agency used my legal name, Nicola, again to show I was European. In Greece, I was called Nikki, to show I was American. People love anything that's not the norm.

At the "old" age of twenty-one, my first assignment took me to Shanghai, China—a vibrant city that was an entirely new world to me with its busy streets, distinctive cuisine, and models from all over the world. What a wake-up call! I thought I was a pretty good model, but I soon realized I was much less experienced than the other girls. To make up for what I considered a lack of experience, I decided to control the only thing I knew how and get even thinner—I ate practically nothing. My weight dropped fast. Apparently, being super-thin was the ticket, because my career really took off.

After Shanghai, I moved back to Colorado and got a job doing marketing for a wellness company. I loved the work, and I picked up bits and pieces of a nutritional puzzle that I would put together much later. I also

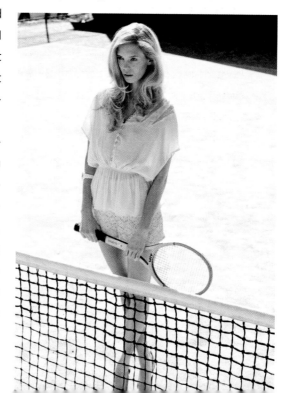

gained back all the weight I had lost. But this was a good thing. I felt much more relaxed about my body because I was happy at home with my friends and family in the Colorado mountains.

Within a year, I got wanderlust, resurrected my modeling career, and headed off to Sydney, Australia, where I found myself moving from house to house, trying to meet friends, get along with roommates, and keep myself busy during off times. It was an amazing place to be, but also extremely isolating. I was lonely, and so I started trying to control what I ate again, limiting myself to miso soup and a few bananas a day.

It was in Sydney that I did my first detox, albeit a pretty hard-core one that lasted six weeks. I cut out all sugar, salt, caffeine, and alcohol and stuck to a ridiculously strict eating plan: plain oatmeal, Greek yogurt, apples, almonds, whole-wheat tortillas, vegetables, and chicken. It was bland indeed, but at least it was somewhat nutritious compared to other diets I'd been on. True to my driven nature, I gave that detox everything I had and dropped from 113 to 103 pounds in six weeks. But I wasn't enjoying my life, and I became a social hermit because it was easier to stay at home than be tempted to stray from my regimen. I thought that eliminating sugar, salt, caffeine, and alcohol would lead to clear skin and sound sleep, but, sadly, it didn't. I was physically and mentally exhausted. But on the upside, that crazy detox gave me my first taste of nutrition and the benefits of eating cleaner foods. I experienced firsthand how you can transform your body when the junk is removed.

In Australia, I lived on beautiful Bondi Beach, where I immersed myself in yoga by going to classes or following videos alone at home. When

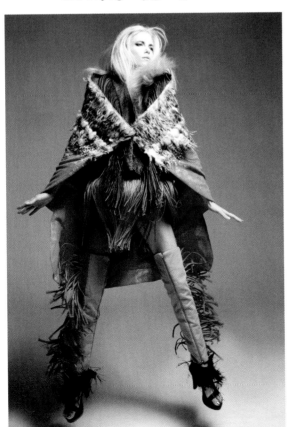

I wasn't modeling, I advanced my practice by teaching myself the Sanskrit names for every pose and their benefits to the body. Each morning, I'd go down to the beach and guide my friends through poses and routines that I had written out on index cards. I was finding my teaching voice and loved giving mini-classes to people who weren't able to practice as intensely as I was. I realized I could take yoga with me as I kept traveling, and that it gave me sanity in the craziest times and places.

One year later, I left Australia

for Seoul, South Korea, where the modeling agencies wanted me to gain weight! So I gobbled down candy bars as quickly as I could buy them. It was as if I'd been given permission to eat whatever I wanted, but on one condition: I could only gain weight in very specific places on my body, such as my lower thighs, but not my upper ones. I didn't gain the weight where they wanted, so I was rejected for some jobs and sent on. I was overwhelmed with headaches every morning, as well as my ever-present acne, constant bloating and constipation, and fear and insecurity about where my life was going and what I was doing with it.

Oh—and on top of everything else, I suffered from insomnia. For seven years, I took prescription sleeping pills. Trust me, I tried *everything* else: chamomile tea, deep breathing, meditation CDs, melatonin, putting my phone and computer away and reading, not reading, getting out of bed when I couldn't sleep, and many more tips that were recommended.

Through it all, I remained in constant pursuit of the ideal body, driven by the need to be skinny or perfect or both. I was never concerned about my inner health or my mental health—only about my physical appearance. I didn't realize that being thin did not actually make me feel good about myself—that sweating like crazy from cardio and starving myself weren't the answers.

Eventually, I became more social and started living the "glamorous" life that went along with modeling. I went out most nights. I'd meet people in a bar after a shoot and we'd move on to a club, where I could easily inhale cocktail after cocktail, do shots, and end the night at 6:00 a.m., only to sleep it off and start up the following day. I partied like most college-age kids do, but I also maintained a strong work ethic: I was punctual and polite, and I always did my best. It was an exciting life, and there were plenty of positives. I was always jetting off to faraway places. I was twenty-three and living all over the globe, learning new languages, meeting new people, and doing what I loved. I did shoots for *More* magazine and *Harper's Bazaar* and walked in shows for Giorgio Armani and Louis Vuitton. I worked extremely hard and became the face of some amazing campaigns worldwide.

MY TURNING POINT

In 2011, I modeled my way through six cities: Seoul, Bangkok, Denver, Athens, London, and New York. On one hand, I felt powerful, beautiful, and proud that I had the career I'd always wanted. On the other, I felt isolated and anxious about getting work and needing to gain or lose weight. I barely had time to call my parents or friends back home. My friendships with other models were fleeting, as we were always moving on to the next job or city. My life felt chaotic, upside-down, and out of control.

Finally I hit my breaking point. I was alternating between extreme food restriction and binges. I wasn't sleeping. I started drinking in secret during the day to deal with my depression and loneliness. The more depressed I got, the worse I ate. The worse I ate, the more I drank. I'd wake up in the morning having a food and alcohol hangover, vow to jump on the healthy bandwagon right then and there, and fall prey to the negative feelings and sugar addiction by that evening. The binges would start again that night and result in more restriction the following day. It was a vicious cycle. *Something had to change.*

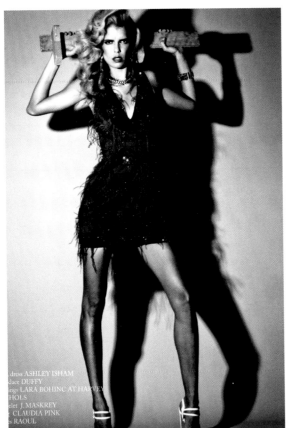

In April 2012, I headed home to Colorado for some much-needed R&R and to literally save my life. I practiced yoga and hiked every day.

While looking in the mirror one day soon after getting home, I realized a very cold, hard truth: that I was literally starving myself to get skinny. And I realized that I couldn't live with myself if I promoted the kind of unhealthy body image that could negatively influence young women. I did not want to spend my life obsessively watching what I ate and counting calories (a habit that always back-fires, as you've probably experienced, too). I knew I had more important things to do. *I wanted to make a difference in the world and help others, not just promote an image of being skinny.*

So I embarked on a journey to find something that worked and made me feel happy. I began educating myself about nutrition and fitness, and I even signed up for a triathlon. I started looking up healthy recipes online, in my mother's cookbooks, and on Instagram. My goal was to eat delicious, nutritious meals that satisfied me so that I wouldn't binge. Deep down, I knew that this, coupled with spending time with loving family and friends, would help me heal.

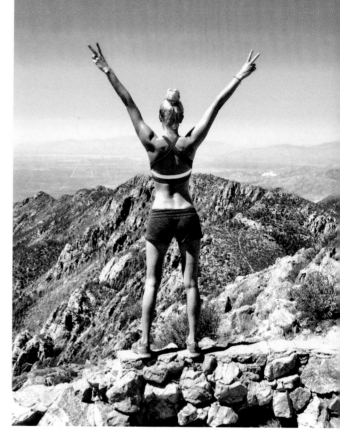

After a month in Colorado and really starting to understand how happy I could be with a healthier lifestyle, I headed back to London, where I realized I wanted to get a regular job and model on the side. I needed stability. I also took courses in raw foods, healthy cooking, sports nutrition, and nutrition for everyday living, both online and at schools in London (and later getting certified as a health coach and yoga teacher). Slowly I taught myself how to take care of my body, mind, and soul. I came to realize that my old lifestyle had taken a piece of me away—and by learning more about the impact of nutrition, I was able to get that piece back. Along the way, I realized that I preferred a different type of fun, one that involved educating and taking care of myself.

Now, I didn't change overnight. There is no such thing as deciding to radically alter your lifestyle 100 percent and never falling back into old habits. Even though I had already experienced the biggest turning point in life, it was not an easy battle. Making changes can be scary. Sometimes you have to say goodbye to unsupportive friends or family members, change jobs, or even move. It can push your strength to the limits.

But when you start to feel how you are truly meant to feel, healthy from the inside out, beautiful, happy, and like you are meant to be here, it's all worth it.

As I became more and more fascinated with food and fitness, my work life was taking a nosedive. I had been working full-time for a few months when suddenly I was let go. Once again, I didn't have enough money to pay my rent and was feeling uncertain about the future. I found myself falling back into restrictive and binge habits to try to control what was happening on the outside. After two months of fruitlessly searching for jobs, I decided that I wanted to take a leap and really commit to a career in health and wellness. I didn't know what it would be, how I would make money, or where to start. I had a small amount of money saved up, just enough to pay rent for a few months, and modeled on the side as I sorted out what my new company would look like. I began blogging about the recipes I had developed, and my Instagram account grew by the day. At the time it was around 3,000 followers who I gained by posting recipes and motivational posts and answering people's questions.

Then came the holiday season. I once again fell into bad habits, drinking heavily into the night, waking up late, and then doing it all over again. I was living a double life, becoming a vocal advocate of healthy living while trashing my body with alcohol, late-night dinners, and restricting and bingeing. By Christmas, I was miserable—bloated, lethargic, and downright sick from weeks of partying. My skin had lost its glow, and I was breaking out badly. My energy levels were nonexistent; the only way I managed to get through each day was by drinking lots of coffee. All of this in two months! I was ashamed of myself. Once again, something had to change. *I needed to clean my body and mind, and quick!*

I looked all over to find a detox that I could start right then and there. I was ready, willing, and extremely eager to start feeling better. But all I found were plans advocating juicing, smoothies, ones that cost almost as much as my rent, meat-heavy diets without many vegetables, or unhealthy calorie restriction. I didn't have the time or money to detox for a long time, and I definitely didn't want to starve myself, because we've seen where that led!

There had to be a better way.

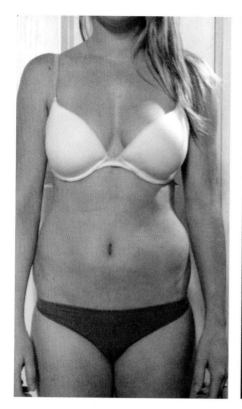
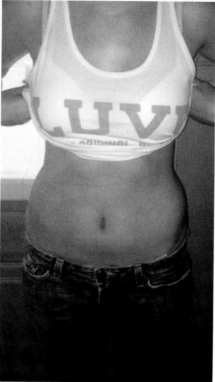

CLEAN FOODS REVEALED

Through all of my courses and self-study, I learned that there are many different fruits, vegetables, and other plant-based foods that have excellent detoxifying properties when eaten as whole foods: beets; cruciferous vegetables such as cauliflower, cabbage, and broccoli; quinoa; apples; berries; almonds; spinach; avocados; tomatoes; legumes; and others. I was certain that these foods, combined with certain herbs and spices, could form the basis of a detox plan that would cleanse the body quickly, taste delicious, and provide superior nutrition.

I also delved into digestive health and, from multiple sources and research, discovered that the body best digests raw, fresh foods early in the day and digests cooked foods better later in the day. This knowledge was imperative to detoxification. *The body can't properly detox unless it can properly digest.*

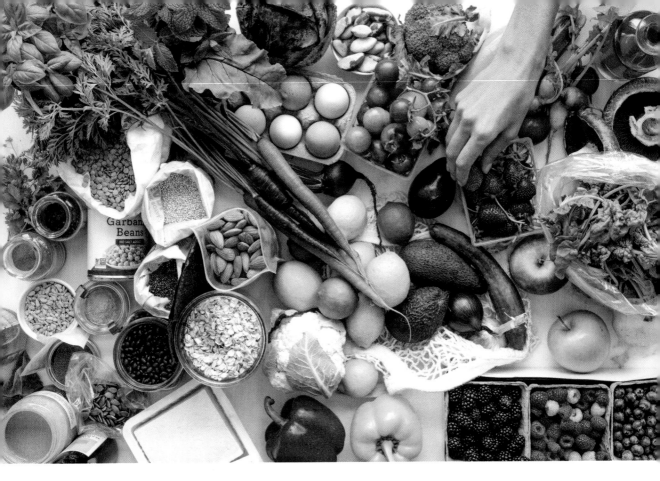

As I refined the cleanse, I made sure that it provided the daily requirements of macronutrients—protein, fats, and carbohydrates—while supplying ample amounts of calcium, iron, magnesium, and other vital nutrients the body needs. I also had to do some extensive trial and error, experimenting with fruits and vegetables that produced the very best results. Bananas, for example, were out, because they were too starchy and less fibrous, while berries were in, because they're low in starch and high in fiber.

I knew I was onto something: no other cleanse out there had you eat meals timed according to optimal digestive functioning. Nor did many focus on clean, wholesome foods that satisfied you.

At the time, all the existing cleanses and diets out there focused on restricting calories like crazy, drinking only juices or smoothies, or eating bland foods. None even delved into the cleansing power of herbs and spices. Using my nutritional knowledge, I knew that I wanted to create a plan that anyone could do—one that would be easy to follow, leave you feeling amazing, and not take over your life for more than a few days. To me, a five-day plan was perfect. It could be started on a Monday, right after a weekend, and finished on a Friday, right before a weekend. I could do anything for just five days!

During this process, I partnered with London-based nutritionist Jill Swyers and registered dietician Helen Phandis to ensure that my calorie and macronutrient calculations were correct. I also wanted to see if there were any alternatives that should be implemented for better digestion, and if there were appropriate substitutions for those who couldn't eat certain foods.

In the beginning, I created this cleanse only for myself, because I hated dieting so much and I didn't want to do any crazy, restrictive program ever again. But it became so much more. I realized I could nourish myself, physically and emotionally, with real, plentiful foods and satisfying flavors. I knew that what I created could help lots of people, not just myself.

The 5-Day Real Food Detox was born.

A PREVIEW

Why is that the name of my plan? Because my detox is built from a huge variety of whole foods—foods that are considered "clean," meaning fresh, natural, nutrient-dense, and free of chemicals, additives, pesticides, and preservatives. I turned all these clean foods into incredibly delicious, satisfying recipes for pancakes, stir-fries, hummus, sushi rolls, and more.

That's right. On my detox, you eat delicious, chewable foods throughout the day while cleansing your system of toxins at the same time. And not one meal a day, but five meals that consist of nutritionally alive ingredients put together in easy-to-follow meal plans. Every part of it works together to maximize the detoxing effects and produce results rapidly.

I started posting about my cleanse on Instagram, not as an income stream, but out of a desire to help people get healthier. I quickly discovered that people wanted my nutritional advice. They were literally hungry for it. That's when I took the plan to the next level and started my company and website, www.nikkisharp.com. At the time I began promoting it in early January 2012, I had just reached ten thousand followers on Instagram and the number of people downloading my ebook was extraordinary. It seemed as though everyone was in the same place as me: wanting to cleanse his or her body with a *real foods* detox, and no more gimmicks!

My readers and fans love the results: you can lose around a pound a day—*you really can*—and perhaps even more, depending on your starting weight. You'll also feel and look totally reenergized. I have received hundreds and hundreds of emails from people sharing their results, proving time and time again that this detox really works.

Since I've been eating more nutritiously, my previous health problems have vanished. Once and for all, my skin has cleared up and truly glows now, although I still break out now and then like everyone else. My headaches are gone and I no longer take any form of stomach medicine. One of the most profound changes I've experienced is that I'm finally sleeping properly for the first time in nine years. I feel so much better now, and it shows to everyone who has seen my photos and videos or met me in person. And I know that if I'm not feeling good, it's because either I have let stress get to me or I'm not eating as cleanly as usual.

I love being healthy, but I still believe in moderation. I will never tell you to cut out things in your life, only to add other, healthier options. By doing this, as you will see on this cleanse, it becomes a habit that you stick to because you *want* to, because you feel and look so darn good!

I've experienced firsthand the angst and guilt that so many people feel in connection to their weight, and all the torture they put themselves through with yo-yo dieting, emotional eating, and fighting with their bodies to get thin. And I've helped my readers and followers overcome these problems. My philosophy is that there is more to nutrition than just dieting and restricting food. Good nutrition is there to enhance your energy, your inner and outer beauty, and your overall quality of life.

I encourage people to strive to become *healthy*, not skinny. The 5-Day Real Food Detox is an important and positive step in that direction.

People who embark on my cleansing adventure are surprised by what happens, even from the very first day. They're amazed at how full they feel. Sometimes they can't even eat all the food—all that *real* food! Then, after five days, when all that weight miraculously falls off and they feel so rejuvenated, they are thrilled, excited, and motivated to continue on their journey by following my Sharp Lifetime Diet, which I cover in this book, too. But don't take it from me: you'll read some of their incredible testimonials in the following pages.

So why starve yourself to get lean and healthy when you can do it in a natural way by actually eating the food that your body wants and needs?

Start my 5-Day Real Food Detox and bid farewell to the bulges and health issues that have been bothering you for so long. Toss aside the foods that have been polluting your body, harming your health, and making you fat, and eat what Mother Nature has provided. Eat clean, and you'll start feeling better about life immediately. You'll overcome issues when you start eating this way, I promise. Look—health, happiness, and fulfillment are yours for the taking. And you deserve all three.

Are you ready to meet a hot, happy new you in just five days? Let's go!

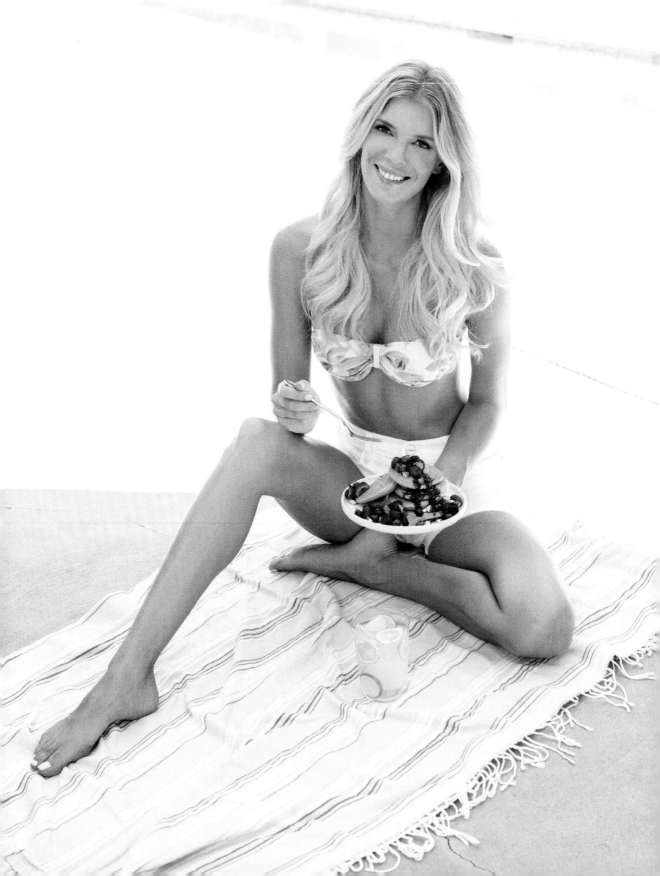

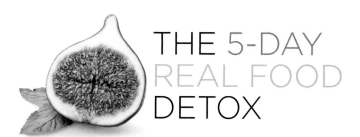

THE 5-DAY
REAL FOOD
DETOX

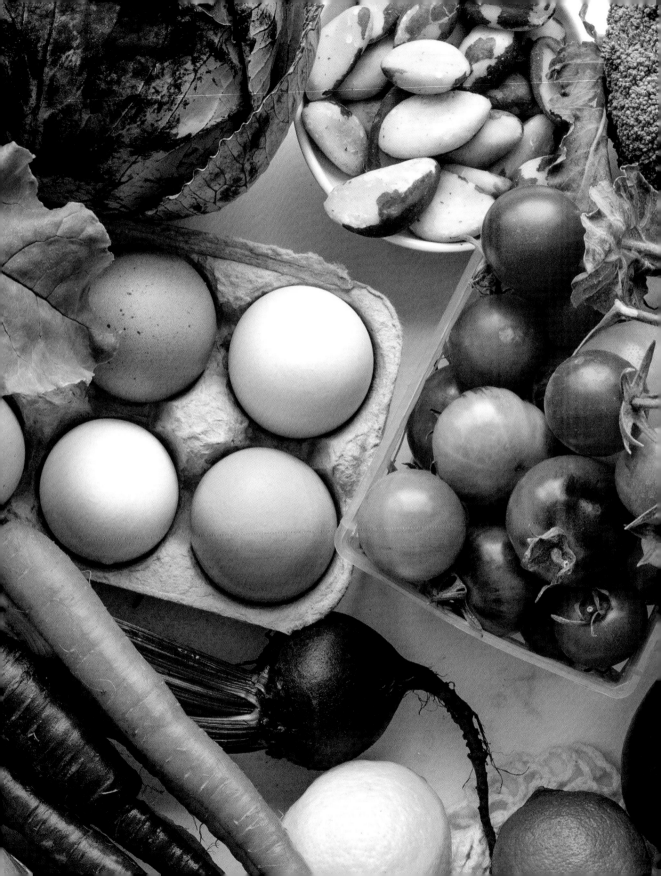

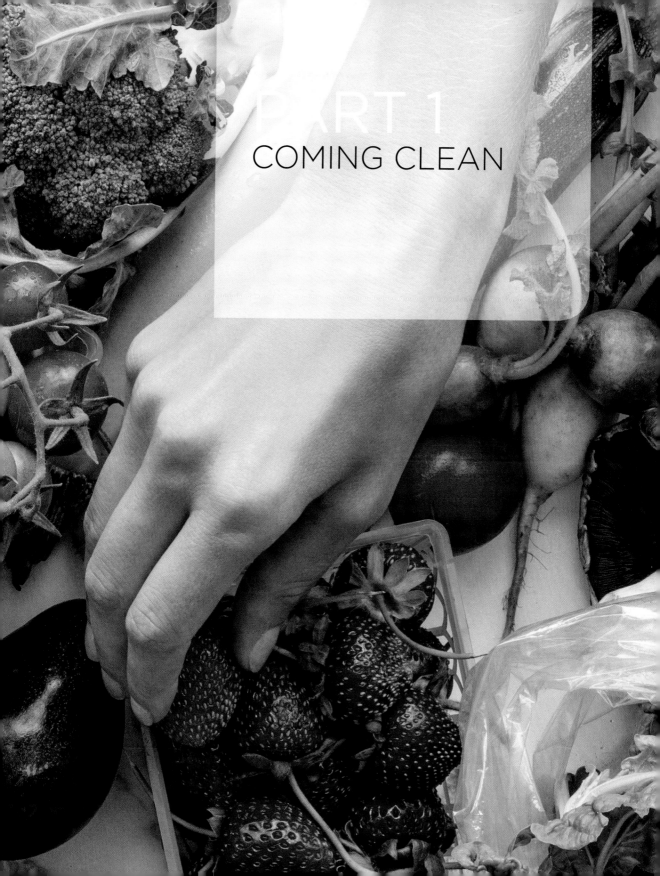

PART 1
COMING CLEAN

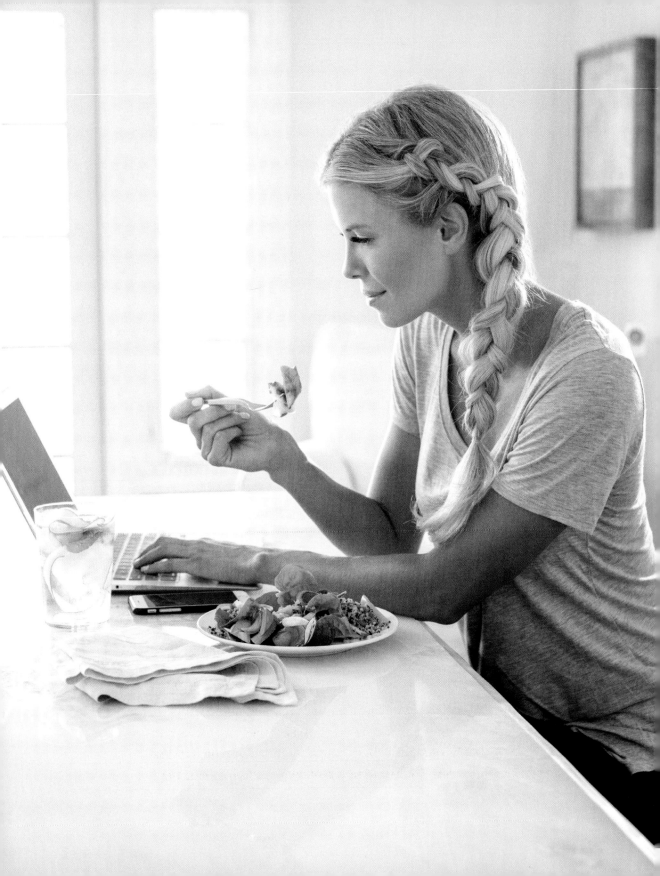

CHAPTER 1

DETOXING WITH CLEAN FOOD

I lost 11 pounds in five days by doing this cleanse, and I'm continuing to drop weight because it taught me how to eat. For the first time in about a year, I put my jeans on . . . and I was so comfortable. I learned that it is not about living one day at a time, but living one decision at a time, and if I'm strong and sharp, I will see results and be happier with myself.

—Rhiana

The world, it seems, is having a love affair with detoxing. It's in vogue simply because it *works*, whether the regimen lasts three, ten, or twenty-one days. Most people who try one report weight loss, clearer skin, reduced bloating, and a rise in energy levels. In fact, in a recent survey of naturopathic doctors in the United States, 92 percent reported using detoxes to treat their patients. The most common reasons they cited were environmental exposure to toxins, general cleansing, preventive healthcare, digestive problems, aches and pains, inflammation, fatigue, and weight loss. It sounds like detoxing is clearly good for us—but why?

DETOXIFICATION—HOW IT WORKS

Detoxification is the cleansing of toxins from the body. By "toxins," I'm talking about the pesticides, artificial hormones, additives, and preservatives with which our food is treated, as well as the excess sugar, alcohol, caffeine, tobacco, pharmaceutical drugs, air pollution, bacteria, and viruses to which our bodies are routinely exposed—either by our own choices or through the environment.

Our food is one of the worst offenders—and it is the one that we have the most control over. But here's the challenge: over the last century, food has become mass produced, mass prepared, and mass consumed, and much of it is of very poor quality as a result. The reasons are many: depleted soils, chemical fertilizers, and the indiscriminate use of pesticides on crops. Other problems that affect food quality include premature harvesting, artificial ripening, genetic engineering, and long transportation times from the source to the store—all of which diminish the nutrients in the food. To make matters worse, a lot of our food is subject to freezing, canning, and irradiation (exposed to radiation to control spoilage and eliminate food-borne germs). And you wonder why your skin breaks out and you don't have any energy?

I once read that we don't eat our food as much as our food eats us. In other words, our food doesn't just supply us with nutrients anymore; it has also become a receptacle for toxins. According to the American Academy of Environmental Medicine, there are some ninety thousand chemicals commonly circulating, many of which may produce chemical sensitivities, with results ranging from allergies to chronically poor health.

Think about pesticides, too: they are so harmful that workers who spray them on the food we eat are required to wear head-to-toe protective gear, as well as gas masks to prevent ingestion and exposure. Those same pesticide-laden fruits and veggies end up in our grocery stores— yet no one warns us to suit up for protection!

Fortunately, the body detoxifies itself naturally. In fact, our bodies are designed to cope with toxins, and usually they do pretty well. The problems arise either when you take in more garbage than your body can handle via junk food, alcohol, smoking, pollution, and so forth, or when your organs in charge of detoxification cannot carry out their jobs as well as they should. Over time, toxins can accumulate in fat cells, in the nervous system, in the bones and soft tissues, and in various other organs and tissues of the body.

Another problem is that there are certain substances not so easily forced out by the body's natural detoxification processes. These include POPs (persistent organic pollutants) and some metals. POPs have been used in the past, as well as currently, as pesticides. They are likely to congregate in fat tissue and can take years to break down. Girls who have been exposed tend to start their periods much earlier than is considered normal because POPs disrupt the function of hormones. For girls who start menstruating at a young age, there are physical and psychological stigmas: breast development (which can make them look stockier than their peers and contributes to their becoming sexually active earlier than others), PMS, weight gain, and embarrassment. There may be scary long-term effects, too. The *New England Journal of Medicine* has reported that the earlier a girl develops breasts, the earlier she might develop breast cancer.

When chemicals can't break down fast enough or the body's processes can't keep up with intake, you can develop a range of symptoms from weight gain, vague aches and pains, headaches, dull skin, acne, lack of energy, insomnia, constipation, and bloating to cellulite, joint pain, depression, and severe fatigue. As if these aren't enough reasons to detox, a buildup of toxins is also associated with diseases such as fibromyalgia, Parkinson's, Alzheimer's, and cancer, just to name a few. All of these are pretty concrete reasons why we should periodically cleanse our bodies with nutritious foods and beverages—and our minds with positive thoughts and emotions.

Do You Need to Detox?

You may still be thinking, why detox? Maybe you already live a pretty healthy lifestyle and only need to make a few tweaks to get fully on track. Or maybe you need to make some big changes.

Either way, I'm not here to judge; rather, I can help guide you to making a few simple choices that will benefit you greatly. And as far as I'm concerned, clean food is the ultimate feel-good, look-great fuel. When you put junk into your body, you feel like junk. When you eat well, you feel well.

Take this brief survey to see if your body can benefit from a clean food detox. Read the following statements, and put a check mark next to the ones that apply to your life. Be honest. Your answers shouldn't reflect your ideal way of living or where you were a year ago. They should describe where you are now.

1. I eat meat more than three times a week.

2. I experience skin breakouts at least once a week.

3. My skin breaks out easily and I am ashamed of it often.

4. I eat fruits and vegetables no more than once a day.

5. I am often constipated.

6. I get sick more often than I would like.

7. I cannot function until I have at least one coffee or energy drink.

8. I smoke socially, when drinking, or when alone.

9. I often have trouble sleeping.

10. I feel like my hair is dull or doesn't have any life to it.

11. I frequently feel bloated.

12. I eat dairy products, such as cheese, cream cheese, milk, cream, or half-and-half at least once a day.

13. I feel most energetic after 5:00 p.m.

14. I often feel like I have very little energy.

15. I drink alcoholic beverages every day, or never during the week but have several drinks on the weekend.

16. I have a big sweet tooth and eat several sugary foods throughout the week.

17. I live in an area of high pollution or smog (such as a city).

18. I often feel stressed.

19. I often sit in traffic or inside a building all day.

20. I exercise once or twice a week or not at all.

21. I eat packaged foods, including sandwiches, sodas, crackers, chips, dips, and desserts, at least three times a week.

If three or more of these statements describe you, a detox will really help you find your way. Remember, it's not about losing weight or just eating better; it's a whole shift toward feeling better about life, yourself, and your goals. Put another way, it can be the first step you take toward resetting your body and mind. And, considering the huge number of chemicals to which we are exposed, I'd say detoxing is important for everyone.

THE ORGANS OF DETOXIFICATION

Although every cell in the body has a role in detoxification, the major players are the liver, kidneys, digestive tract, skin, and lungs. Here's how they work. The liver alone churns out thirteen thousand different detoxifying enzymes, small proteins that act as catalysts to speed up the chemical reactions in our bodies. Nothing goes on in the body without enzymes; in fact, life cannot exist without them. They are indispensable for digestion, a well-running immune system, and detoxification. Most enzymes work by taking apart matter. For instance, digestive enzymes break down the meal you just ate into its smallest components. Antioxidant enzymes dismantle disease-causing free radicals. And liver enzymes break down all sorts of toxins, from drugs to alcohol to pollutants, then eliminate them from the body as harmless by-products, filtered out by the kidneys and digestive system.

The kidneys rely on liver enzymes to convert toxins into water-soluble substances that can be eliminated. The digestive system gets rid of contaminants by excreting undigested food so that it does not build up and cause digestive problems. Taking good care of our intestines and colon with high-fiber food is the best way to keep the digestive system detoxed.

The skin is key, too, because it is our largest organ. We sweat out waste (including heavy metals) from our pores, which is why drinking lots of water helps keep your complexion clear and why you'll quickly notice glowing skin when you cut out the junk. Working out is a great way to detox, too, because it makes you perspire. If an injury keeps you from exercising, you can still stimulate your sweat glands with periodic trips to the sauna. (But be sure to drink plenty of water after steam-cleaning yourself!)

In addition, our lungs expel carbon dioxide and other waste products and work best when we breathe unpolluted air. If we don't have clean air, we can get very sick. Research indicates that many respiratory illnesses, such as asthma and Legionnaire's disease, are the direct result of breathing unclean air in our homes, workplaces, and schools. And a large body of research suggests that inhaling airborne particles discharged by vehicles, factories, and power plants can prompt heart problems and aggravate respiratory diseases in susceptible people, leading to perhaps sixty thousand premature deaths annually in the United States.

Eating clean foods, particularly fruits and vegetables high in vitamins C and E, protects our lungs from pollutants. Deep breathing through yoga or meditation is another way to help them out. The more oxygen there is in your lungs, the more effectively you'll expel the bad stuff, so make sure to allow a little time every day to take some deep breaths. These will also oxygenate your blood for more efficient delivery of nutrients to cells and tissues, clearing out all the CO_2 to make room for fresh air in the body. I'll talk more about breathing techniques in Chapter 6.

Note from Nikki: Can I Detox If I Smoke?

Speaking of lungs, what if you're a smoker? Smoking can be incredibly hard to give up, and I'm not here to say that you need to start that journey right now. The good news? You absolutely can and should detox even if you smoke—I know you'll still see great benefits. What I will suggest, though, is try to reduce your habit if possible, even by one cigarette a day. Not so bad? Then try cutting out two.

I know that smoking helps a lot of people skip meals in order to lose weight. But I want you to follow the cleanse to the letter, without skipping meals, changing them, or substituting a cigarette when you get a craving. Learning to deal with cravings the natural way will not only improve your health but also show you how strong your willpower can truly be, and you'll feel more in control in all areas of your life. You might not even need cigarettes as much once your body begins to feel lighter and more energized. Just remember to drink lots of water, especially infused water, and to stimulate your palate with the recommended spices and herbs.

And believe it or not, one of the most effective ways to overcome smoking is not only by trying to quit but also by infusing your body with green vegetables, particularly in the form of green smoothies. There are a couple of reasons this works. For one thing, people often confuse hunger with the desire to smoke. So instead of reaching for a cigarette, reach for a green smoothie (it will fill you up and ease your hunger), or go for something to keep your mind busy, like crunching on an apple. If the cravings get bad, try smelling and playing with spearmint toothpicks. Also, smokers tend to be deficient in vitamin C. The green leafy vegetables in a green smoothie are loaded with the vitamin C you need. I've seen the worst of smokers kick their habit this way. Smoking is not an easy habit to kick, so what I want you to take away is that you are on a journey and it's okay if you cannot quit right now.

TYPES OF DETOXES

There are many different types of detoxes, so be careful to avoid the extreme, unhealthy ones. Perhaps you've already tried one, whether it's a trendy fasting diet, a liquid cleanse, or a fat-melting pill (yeah, right!).

Many of these can be harmful, leading to an imbalance of nutrients, in-filtrating your bloodstream with toxic substances, slowing down your metabolism, and causing your weight to yo-yo.

Plus, a lot of them are based on rigid protocols, allowing you only juice, smoothies, water, or raw foods—and I have strong opinions on each of these.

Juice Detoxes

I'm a huge advocate of juicing. It can be an effective way to flood your body with nutrients that you might not otherwise get. Used in non-Western medicine for hundreds of years, it can also cleanse your body, eliminate bloating, ward off cravings, increase energy, clear up skin, and even treat serious diseases. Not to mention that it's all the rage right now, with new juice bars and home delivery services popping up to capitalize on the trend.

So juicing is the best thing ever, right? Well, *not exactly.* Where people go wrong is by drinking too many fruits and not enough vegetables. Fruit juice—even if you make it yourself—is a highly concentrated source of sugar. Yes, it's natural sugar, accompanied by vitamins, minerals, and phytochemicals. But it can have a surprisingly high calorie count. More important, what's missing from juice is fiber. Without fiber, the body absorbs sugar more quickly, triggering a rapid increase in blood sugar levels and impeding metabolism. Also, we need fiber to assist our bowels in healthy elimination. Some juice cleanses advise you to supplement with psyllium husk powder, or to schedule colonics or enemas to assist with bowel movements. Any protocol that requires an extra step (like a colonic) in order to use the toilet is not a healthy way to cleanse.

And *please* stay away from commercial fruit juice, which is often laced with refined sugars such as table sugar (sucrose) or high-fructose corn syrup, neither of which contains the nutrients found in natural fruit juices. A report published in the *American Journal of Public Health* in 2012 noted, "Excessive fruit juice consumption is associated with in-creased risk for obesity. Moreover, there is recent scientific evidence that sucrose consumption without the corresponding fiber, as is commonly present in fruit juice, is associated with the metabolic syndrome, liver injury, and obesity." Bottom line: the calories you drink as fruit juice are more likely to show up on the scale than the calories you chew as actual fruits—plus lead to additional health problems.

Juices also lack protein, which we need to maintain our beautiful, body-defining muscle. In fact, within the first two days of a juice cleanse (if you last that long), your body is coerced into burning precious muscle for fuel. Nutrient deficiencies interfere with detoxification and starve out helpful gut bacteria. On my plan, you'll get all the protein you need— but more on that later.

What's more, all-juice detoxes, particularly vegetable-based ones, are extremely low in calories, so your body goes into panic mode and clings to its fat stores to avert starvation. Even if you do lose a few pounds, it's mostly water weight. Your brain also sends up an SOS to halt some processes to conserve fuel. I'm talking about hormone production and healing, both of which are vital to your health—anything that cuts them off is not going to make you feel better. Doing a juice cleanse can have the effect of slowing down your metabolism and in extreme cases lead to the onset of an eating disorder. It's important to recognize these negative side effects during a juice cleanse.

Many people swear by juice fasts, and I'm not here to say they are incorrect. What works for some won't work for others. Juicing is a beautiful method to inundate your body with nutrients, but rather than drink juice all week long to the exclusion of clean solid food, try enjoying it as a nutrient-loaded snack. If you really want to try it, do a one-day green juice fast to give your body a healthy kick start. Anything longer than a day won't teach you the necessary habits to eat nutritiously over the long term.

Smoothie Detoxes

What I love about smoothies is that they can really help you beat cravings for good. The reason is that they contain fiber, which makes you feel full. Whenever someone tells me she isn't confident that she'll succeed on my detox, I always recommend adding one of my green smoothie recipes for one to two weeks before trying the full detox. It conquers cravings by creating fullness, boosts energy, and brightens up skin.

Although this is the healthiest of all the fad cleanses we'll discuss, it can be hard to maintain. Who wants to drink smoothies for days on end? This can be boring and too restrictive, possibly leading to binge-ing and weight gain once you stop the smoothie diet. I don't promote this method because it still doesn't teach you how to *eat*. I've found that when people do this type of detox, they do see results and feel amaz-ing, but have a hard time when life kicks back in and they have to go to restaurants, resist treats at work, and make dinner for their family. Smoothies are a great complement to a healthy diet; however, I don't think they are the best for a cleanse.

It's also tough if you live in a place where it isn't warm all the time. Ask people in the middle of a cold winter if they want a smoothie or a bowl of soup, and the answer is almost always the latter. We need dif-ferent foods to support us in different seasons, and in winter, something that cools the body will not aid in digestion, help your metabolism, or keep you satisfied as much as a warming or grounding food will.

Bottom line: I do include a smoothie on my cleanse, but you get to enjoy it alongside many other delicious foods.

Water Fasting

And then there's water fasting and its variations, such as the Master Cleanse, which incorporates lemon juice and cayenne pepper. Celebri-ties sometimes do it—and tweet about it—to slim down quickly for a film role, but they have a team of doctors following along. It's not ter-ribly realistic, is it? Fine if you're a monk contemplating spirituality atop a mountain somewhere, but less fine if you're a mom with a couple of kids who think french fries are a food group.

Water fasting can be harmful because it can trigger muscle break-down. Blood levels of ammonia and nitrogen rise as muscle breaks down, resulting in nausea or weakness, according to a Swedish study published in the journal *Metabolism*.

The bottom line: skip water fasts. Your body needs nutrients from real food to carry out detoxification, fight infections, and keep your metabolism ticking along nicely.

Tea-toxes

You may have seen certain celebrities promoting tea-toxes on social media lately. Now let's be real: a tea-tox is a water fast by another name, and it's still a bad idea in my book. The ingredients in some teas, such as green tea, mint, fennel, and cinnamon, can be very healthy, reducing bloating and appetite and increasing metabolism and energy. But who wants to drink tea all day to the exclusion of delicious food?

Also, in most tea-toxes, the "secret ingredient" is senna, a plant native to India and China. It is used to relieve constipation and can be found in many teas, some of which I actually promote if you occasionally need a natural laxative. However, when you are drinking three to five servings a day, your body begins to shed water weight, not actual fat, which means you will gain that back as soon as you start eating normally again. Excess senna, like any laxative, can also create a laxative dependency in your body, leaving you unable to have a bowel movement without it.

Also, when you drink only liquids all day long, you're pretty much starving your body. That's because liquids, unlike solid foods, do very little to activate hunger-suppressing hormones. What's more, liquid diets are all about restriction. I don't know about you, but there's nothing like banning something to make me want it more. It's fine to drink these teas in moderation, but only as a supplement to a clean, healthy diet. It's far healthier to eat high-fiber fruits and vegetables, which promote healthy bowel activity while providing your body with energy for workouts and daily life—and fill you up so that you don't feel like bingeing.

My verdict: any type of all-liquid approach, whether it's juice, water, or a liquid shake, freaks me out a bit. Whenever I've tried one, I felt ridiculous drinking my food all day—and I was always "hangry." All I could think about was all the glorious food I wanted to eat. I mean, how do you come off a liquid diet and not lick your plate clean the first chance you get?

Raw Food Detoxes

I've also tried a 100 percent raw food plan, and it wasn't for me. After a week, I realized that I wasn't eating as nutritiously as I normally would, because I tended to overeat nuts, seeds, and dried fruit, and skimp on fresh fruits and vegetables. I found that I was constantly bloated and

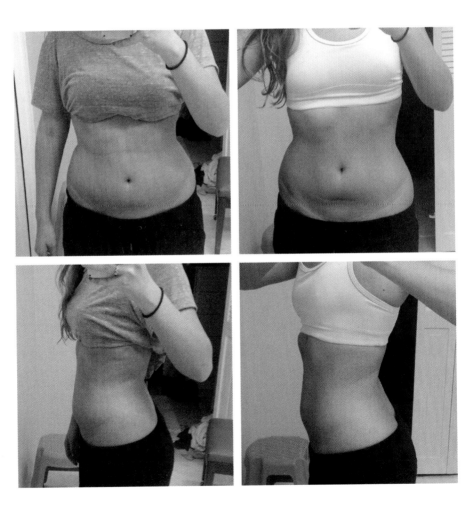

lacked the high energy levels that many people report by eating raw foods. I also felt cold all the time and never felt satisfied. I learned this is due to having a weak digestive system, which is actually very common. All this means is that your body has a harder time processing the raw fiber in uncooked foods, therefore leading to less nutrient absorption and lack of digestion. It's nothing to be worried about; it just means that eating primarily raw foods doesn't work as well for your body. It was by trial and error and listening to my own body that I realized that eating a *balance* of raw and cooked meals was the answer, not only for my digestive system but for my palate as well. Cooked foods just satisfy me more.

Don't get me wrong. I'm not against raw foods; in fact, they're absolutely essential to a healthy body. I'm just against eating raw foods *only*. I adhere to, and aim to teach others, a more harmonious way of eating. Everyone is an individual, so we all have different foods that will nourish us. Like all things in life, balance and moderation are key.

Now that we've cleared that up, I hope you're thinking, *Isn't there a better way to cleanse your body?*

Absolutely!

THE 5-DAY REAL FOOD DETOX: OVERVIEW

And that's a plan based on *real* food rather than dousing your body with juices or smoothies, drinking only water all day, or abstaining from solids—all of which can result in serious problems. My cleanse is one of the few out there that allows you to eat a wide variety of nutrient-dense foods throughout the day, with simple recipes that anyone can prepare and follow. Real food means food that comes from Mother Nature: vegetables, fruits, grains, legumes, nuts, seeds, herbs, and spices.

These foods encourage detoxification, primarily because their nutrients support the function of the organs directly involved in cleansing the body. Unlike most detoxes and diets, my plan also teaches you how to eat afterward for lifelong success. No more ups and downs. It's time to finally lose that weight and get healthy and happy once and for all. And you'll do it with a few simple tools.

> ## DETOXIFIED!
>
> I started my weight loss journey in October at 234 pounds because I realized I wanted to live a healthier life and feel good about the skin I'm in. I started eating better, working out, gaining muscle, and toning up. I even signed up for my first half-marathon next March. I reached a plateau of about 222 pounds at one point, so I started the cleanse. Today I weighed in at 214.7 pounds. This detox showed me that clean eating will help me reach my goals. I'll continue to incorporate a lot of the recipes into my life after the five days are up. I've been shown a new way of fueling my body and mind!
>
> —Sofie R.

HOW TO USE THE DETOX

The idea is simple. You'll eat a variety of plant-based foods, deliciously prepared, five times a day—all for just five days. You'll cut out foods containing harmful chemicals, while flushing out impurities by drinking plenty of water.

This cleanse is not a diet. Diets are typically followed for a certain period of time, after which the dieter often returns to poor eating habits. My cleanse, on the other hand, is meant to kick-start a program of healthy eating that lasts long after the five days are over. I see no point in detoxing for several days, then cramming your body full of toxins again. Use this as your entry into a new world of eating and living. It will:

- Jump-start weight loss in just five days. Check out the real-life results throughout this book. Amazing, aren't they?
- Help you drop those stubborn, final pounds if you've been dieting for a while, plus smash through any frustrating weight-loss plateaus.
- Give you a youthful glow. Toxic accumulation can result in skin prob-

lems (from rashes to acne to wrinkles to under-eye circles) and brittle hair and nails. When you cleanse with clean foods, you support the body's detox organs and neutralize and eliminate toxins from the inside out. A clean diet will also clear up pimples, skin reactions, and acne, and even minimize cellulite.

- Solve your energy crisis. Toxins cause fatigue and general sluggishness. The cleanse helps eliminate them efficiently so that you'll have renewed energy in a matter of days. Not only will you be kicking all the bad things out of your body, you'll introduce high levels of nutrients to pump you full of energy and keep you feeling great throughout the day—without having to rely on the artificial "ups" you get from caffeine.

- Sharpen your brain. Toxins can burden your brain and lead to foggy thinking. My detox delivers foods that power your brain to do its work. It's a busy organ, and thus prone to cellular stress. Antioxidants to the rescue. These miracle nutrients guard against the oxidation (a destructive process similar to rusting) of brain cells brought on by toxins, and multiple studies provide evidence of this. Researchers at Tufts, for example, reporting in a 2009 issue of the *Journal of Neuroscience*, noted that antioxidants pay a "longevity dividend," particularly in brain health, and that recent studies suggest that eating a diet rich in antioxidants and anti-inflammatory components such as those found in fruits, nuts, vegetables, and spices may reduce age-related brain declines and the risk of developing brain diseases.

- Improve your memory. The brain is 60 percent fat and also needs good fats for peak function. You'll be getting them from olive oil, avocado, nuts, and seeds. The net effect of good nutrition is clearer thinking, improved mood, and sharper memory.

- Give you a psychological boost. Doing the cleanse and changing your nutrition afterward is empowering, not just physically, but mentally. Yes, you *can* do this—and gain the momentum to go on to enjoy greater vitality and health for a lifetime. No more being a slave to binges and thoughts of, "Well, I've already messed my diet up, so I might as well eat the rest of this." You'll gain the willpower to say no when you want, and learn to really savor the foods that do your body good.

- Lead the way to lifelong nutritional changes. This is the gateway to a whole new world of eating and living, where you no longer have to diet, obsess over your body, feel tired and frustrated, and carry the baggage of poor nutrition. Your entire relationship with food will change for the better; food will be your ally, not your enemy. Your experience will be so motivating that you will want to come back to it whenever you're feeling overweight, unattractive, sluggish, or just plain bad. I know you'll want to adopt my after-tox, the Sharp Lifetime Diet, to maintain your results.
- Get you into a smaller size—fast! Let's be realistic: the instant perks of my plan are great, too. Use it to prep for an important weekend event or big date. You'll be able to fit into your bathing suit, wedding dress, tux, prom dress, or any sexy outfit you want. Use it to lose weight gained on vacation or during the holidays, too.

I am forever grateful for the restorative powers of real food, and honored to pass this knowledge on to you, so that you can live your best, healthiest life. Food—pure, natural, and whole—is the first and foremost form of medicine. Without it, few therapies or healing regimens are effective. It fortifies our life force, giving us strength, energy, happiness, and self-renewal—something we've never gotten with a fast-food burger. So why not try something new? Just by picking up this book, you're already on that path. Let me guide you through this journey into finally feeling wonderful about yourself, life, and the food you eat.

CHAPTER 2

WHY IT WORKS
THE METABOLIC DETOX PRINCIPLES

I did your detox last summer and had amazing results: each night I'd retire to bed with no bloating—just a flat stomach! This has never happened before. Since then I have done it about once a month. Your recipes have *so* much flavor and they are so simple. I'm now a quinoa addict!

—Brittany

Nothing can compare to how you'll feel after doing this cleanse. You'll have more energy, a tighter tummy, and a clearer mind, and you'll feel happier. You will glow from within. It's like giving your body a thorough tune-up, and let's face it, we all need one from time to time.

So why does it work so well? You know the old saying, "There's a method to my madness"? Well, there's a method to my cleanse! Whether it's changing your diet, learning unfamiliar ways of thinking, or trying a new exercise routine, you'll always be more successful if you know the reasoning behind it. Gone are the days of people telling you to eat more fruit because "it's good for you," or to not eat carbs after 3:00 p.m. because "you'll gain weight." It's time to educate yourself on why certain actions affect the body and mind, and there are four key principles you should know about.

1. MY DETOX IS PLANT-BASED

Many diets today promote high protein and low-carb/low-fat or some combination of the two. Having tried everything on the market, I've found that the only nutritional plan that ever helps me lose weight, keep it off, reduce cravings, and improve my entire body is a plant-based one.

And my experience has been validated many times over by science. One 2013 study reported that a plant-based (vegan) diet triggered greater weight loss over an eight-week period and six months than did diets that included meat. At the eight-week mark, participants eating vegan lost an average of 8 to 10 pounds, while those on a conventional diet shed 5. At six months, the vegans had peeled off 7 percent of their starting body weight, while the meat-eaters dropped only between 3 and 4 percent.

Plant-based diets work wonders for a few important reasons. First, they improve insulin sensitivity. This simply means that your body is using the hormone insulin properly to help your cells obtain glucose (blood sugar) from your bloodstream for energy. If your cells become insensitive to insulin, they basically snub the hormone when it tries to escort sugar into those cells to be burned for fuel, and that sugar stockpiles in your system, where it can injure blood vessels, tissues, and organs, and get stored as fat, too.

Second, with plant-based diets, you don't have to count calories, points, or grams of anything. It's so easy to get caught up in that minutiae when our real focus should be on the nutritional components of the food. In a plant-based diet, the food you eat is naturally low in calories and fat (although it will contain good amounts of essential fats the body needs). It also dramatically increases your intake of nutrients.

To take advantage of the nutritional power of plants, count colors instead of calories. Make a rainbow on your plate: bright red strawberries, deep green kale, velvety purple eggplant. The more colorful a meal is, the more nutrients it has. I haven't counted calories in years. I'm free from having to work so hard to maintain a fit, healthy figure—and you will be, too.

Third, plant-based diets are loaded with fiber, a great detoxifier. Because your body can't digest fiber, it journeys through the digestive tract collecting harmful substances such as excess fat and toxins and sweeps them out. Without fiber, a lot of this stuff is reabsorbed and recirculated through the body.

People in Western cultures generally do not eat enough fiber, and this is a pretty serious issue. Low-fiber diets can lead to a variety of diseases, including appendicitis, heart disease, diabetes, obesity, and colon cancer. Eating more plant-based fiber—rather than relying on laxatives—is one of the simplest ways you can improve your diet and your health.

Let's open up about something that we don't like talking about: poop. I understand that this subject makes many people uncomfortable, but stick with me. This is an important conversation, because so many people who follow the standard American diet (SAD) experience constipation.

You can tell how well your body's digestive system is working by the number of bowel movements you have daily. There's no right or wrong amount; it's more about what is normal for your body. However, it's considered healthy to have at least one a day. Switch to a plant-based diet, and you may begin going after every meal! That's good, because you'll experience less bloating, feel lighter, and have a flatter tummy.

Fiber also tames your desire to overeat. Fibrous foods such as fruits, vegetables, legumes, nuts, and whole grains provide stomach-filling bulk and stimulate the release of appetite-suppressing hormones. As a result, you get full and are less tempted to reach for seconds. Fiber is awesome because it helps you to lose weight without ever feeling deprived.

High-fiber foods also take longer to chew, so your meals last longer. That's a plus, since it takes about twenty minutes after starting a meal for your body to send signals to your brain that it's full. And, when eaten with other nutrients, fiber slows the rate of digestion, curbing your appetite between meals.

Fiber also helps your body normalize blood sugar levels. After you eat a piece of fruit or a starchy carbohydrate, such as brown rice or

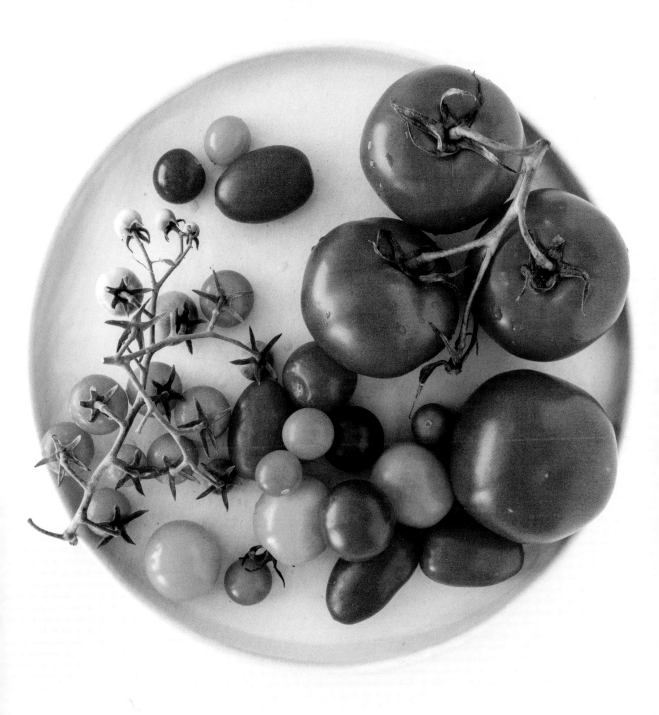

winter squash, your stomach is so busy breaking down the fiber that any sugar is more slowly digested. In other words, it puts the brakes on sugar digestion, so you don't get that quick high and even quicker crash.

I've taken into consideration all these benefits of plant-based nutrition, concentrated into a five-day plan that produces results you'll see and feel. Plants rule the world!

2. THE CLEANSE DEPLOYS TOXIC AVENGERS

Detoxes frequently get criticized because they skimp on vital nutrients. Mine amply supplies the vitamins, minerals, antioxidants, and phytochemicals essential to achieving high-level health. Many have special detox functions, which is why I call them "toxic avengers." Here's a rundown.

Antioxidants

Antioxidants are chemicals found naturally in plant foods. They include beta-carotene and vitamins A and C, along with the mineral selenium. Antioxidants help combat the harmful effects of unstable molecules known as free radicals. Free radicals are chemicals given off during the normal metabolism of food and through general wear and tear on body cells. Infections, junk food, alcohol, sunlight (from both the sun and artificial tanning machines), cigarette smoke, and pollution can all generate them.

Fortunately for our beautiful bodies, free radicals are excreted through urine, sweat, and stool. But in order for elimination to happen, they must first be made water-soluble—which is what antioxidants and other nutrients do. The process of converting these free radicals into a disposable form is an important part of detoxification.

Also, because a proper detox can help banish free radicals, your immune system will be stronger, and you'll have a lower risk of catching the common cold and flu, and possibly reduce your chances of getting cancer and other life-threatening diseases.

Certain vegetables, such as spinach, provide another powerhouse: glutathione. It's technically an amino acid (protein fragment) and the most powerful antioxidant in our bodies. Without glutathione, other antioxidants can't do their jobs to protect our bodies against disease. It detoxifies a wide range of chemicals and boots out toxins that get trapped in fat tissue.

Phytochemicals

Phytochemicals are also found in food, but unlike antioxidants, they're not vitamins or minerals. There are hundreds—and maybe thousands—that occur naturally in plants, and they do some amazing things for our health. For example, they're potent warriors against a major cause of cancer: environmental toxins. These toxins damage our DNA and can switch on cancer-causing genes that would otherwise have remained dormant. Although it's impossible to avoid them altogether, you can arm your body with phytochemicals from food to remove them from your system before they can cause any damage. According to a report published in 2012 in the Polish medical journal *Roczniki Państwowego Zakładu Higieny*, phytochemicals—particularly those found in broccoli, cauliflower, and Brussels sprouts—neutralize chemical threats by optimizing the body's detoxification system, protecting cell membranes, strengthening immunity, and decreasing the risk of cancer. The result is unmatched protection from the unavoidable assaults of modern daily living.

Among the chief phytochemical detoxifiers are:

Succinic acid. A natural chelator, meaning that it combines with, and helps eliminate, heavy metals from the body. This is important, because a heavy metal like mercury, found in certain fish species, can stay in the blood for fifty-seven days, and lead can remain in bones for twenty to thirty *years*. Found in apples and berries.

Chlorophyll. Helps increase levels of oxygen in your blood, and assists in cleansing the body and strengthening your immune system. Found in green leafy vegetables like kale and spinach.

Sulfur. Boosts levels of enzymes that detoxify potential carcinogens, alleviates symptoms of allergies, and improves lung function. Abundant in garlic and onions.

Dithiolethiones. Trigger the formation of an enzyme that makes cancer-causing agents easier to excrete. Found in broccoli.

Glucosinolates. Assist your liver in ridding the body of chemicals, drug residues, and pollutants. They also kill cancer cells and are involved in suppressing the growth of tumors. What's more, there's evidence that glucosinolates can deactivate genes that promote the spread of cancer. Found in cruciferous vegetables such as cauliflower, cabbage, and broccoli.

Sulforaphane. A compound that boosts the activity of detoxification enzymes and antioxidants, it has been found to substantially reduce the risk of many cancers, including some of the deadliest forms, such as cancer of the pancreas, breast, colon, and esophagus. Kale is loaded with it.

Flavonoids. A broad classification of phytochemicals found in fruits, vegetables, and tea. Basically, these are pigments that act as antioxidants, helping to detox free radicals and increasing the activity of liver detoxification enzymes. They give plant foods their vibrant colors. The more reds, oranges, greens, yellows, and blues you put on your plate, the more detoxing properties you are getting.

The B-team. The liver needs additional nutrients for your systems to work well, including vitamins B_2, B_3, B_6, B_{12}, and folic acid. These B vitamins assist the liver in its detoxification activities. Find them in fruits, green leafy vegetables, carrots, cucumbers, onions, legumes, root vegetables, brown rice, and nuts. A related nutrient is lecithin, found in egg yolks. (On the cleanse, you can eat an egg every day if you like.) Lecithin has a lipotropic influence, meaning it accelerates the removal of fat from the liver cells.

These toxic avengers help flush out all sorts of junk, including what scientists call obesogens, chemicals found in meat, dairy, processed sugars, and plastic food and beverage containers that throw our fat-producing hormones out of whack. Obesogens do damage in a couple of ways. They interfere with the release of leptin, the body's natural "I'm full" signal. They prompt the body to store fat. They reprogram cells to become fat cells. And they promote insulin insensitivity. Bottom line: obesogens can accumulate in our bodies, destroying our natural weight-control system and making it nearly impossible to lose those extra pounds.

Scientists have identified many different obesogens in foods and in our environment. I've listed and summarized them in the table below—and suggested how to avoid them.

Fattening Chemicals in Food

THE CHEMICAL	WHERE IT LURKS	HOW TO AVOID IT
Bisphenol A (BPA)	Lining of food cans, plastic bottles, and cash register receipts	Eat organic foods, drink filtered water, and minimize exposure to plastic and food cans made with BPA. Use glass for food storage, and never heat or microwave plastic. Drink out of glass or stainless steel. Cut down on canned foods, particularly acidic ones like tomatoes, which are more apt to absorb the chemicals from the lining.
Fructose	Processed foods, sodas, commercial juices, commercial sweets and desserts	Eat organic foods and avoid any food product containing fructose or high-fructose corn syrup, corn sugar, isolated fructose, or glucose syrup.
Monosodium glutamate (MSG)	Processed foods and foods served in many Asian and ethnic restaurants	Read labels and avoid any foods containing MSG or glutamate. In ethnic restaurants, request that foods be prepared without MSG.
Perfluorooctanoic acid (PFOA)	Microwavable trays and packaging such as those found in popcorn bags and pizza boxes	Avoid these processed foods. Use an air popper for popcorn.

Fattening Chemicals in the Environment

THE CHEMICAL	WHERE IT LURKS	HOW TO AVOID IT
Chlorpyrifos	A pesticide that has been banned for use in homes due to its tendency to cause delayed development in children but is still heavily used in produce crops.	Eat organic foods.

Fattening Chemicals in the Environment

THE CHEMICAL	WHERE IT LURKS	HOW TO AVOID IT
Organotins	Fungicides for crops such as nuts, potatoes, rice, and celery, as well as a toxic substance used in rodent repellents.	Eat organic foods.
Phthalates	Food packaging, laundry products, perfumes, soap, moisturizers, insecticides, and building materials. Can disrupt endocrine levels and result in pregnancy loss and adult infertility.	Use natural cleaning products or make your own, using vinegar diluted in water. Avoid plastics marked #3, and products that list "fragrance" as an ingredient. Eat organic food.
Polychlorinated biphenyls (PCBs)	Pollutants that are produced by the electrical, plastics, pesticide, paper, and other industries. A food source is farm-raised salmon. (Although banned decades ago, PCBs are still in the environment and have been linked to cancer.)	Certain fish species such as shark, swordfish, king mackerel, tilefish, and large tuna steaks may contain PCBs, so consider limiting your intake of these fish. Reduce your use of plastic products.
Polybrominated diphenyl ethers (PBDEs)	Flame retardants used in electrical equipment, construction material, mattresses, and textiles. Food sources include farm-raised salmon, meat, and dairy products. Can cause liver toxicity and impair memory.	Wash your hands frequently. Commit to using PBDE-free products. Eat less meat and dairy; choose wild-caught salmon over the farm-raised variety.
Smoking/nicotine	Tobacco products. Can lead to asthma, type 2 diabetes, lung, mouth, stomach, and kidney cancers.	Don't smoke, even socially! Secondhand smoke should be avoided as much as possible; e-cigarettes are just as bad.

 Note from Nikki: The Cellulite Situation

I can't talk about obesogens, weight gain, and body fat without addressing cellulite, those dreaded dimples that crop up on our thighs and butt. Cellulite develops when the strands of connective tissue that join the fat tissue to the skin get thicker while our skin gets thinner.

Many people think cellulite is just regular, run-of-the-mill fat. It is not. It is a fatty product of toxic waste material—primarily obesogens—and sluggish circulation. Its presence indicates that the body is overloaded with toxins that have been trapped in these areas. When excess fat and toxins form deposits, bulges are created—and voilà, cellulite. Of course, there are other factors involved in cellulite formation, as pointed out in a 2012 review published in the *Journal of the European Academy of Dermatology and*

Venereology: connective tissue weaknesses, hormonal imbalances, blood circulation problems, and genetics. The role of diet in treating cellulite has not been fully explored; all I know is that when I eat nutritious, detoxifying foods, my cellulite is minimized, and I've seen this benefit in my clients, too. Body brushing can also help reduce cellulite, and we'll get into this later in the book.

3. THE CLEANSE RESTORES YOUR ALKALINE-ACID BALANCE

For those of you who barely remember high school chemistry, here's a quick remedial course. The human body works hard 24/7 to maintain the blood's balance of alkaline to acid, known as pH. The letters stand for "power of hydrogen," because pH measures the concentration of hydrogen. The pH scale runs from 1 to 14 and measures the acidity or alkalinity of a substance, including food, blood, and sweat, with lower numbers signifying greater acidity and higher numbers greater alkalinity: 1 to 6.9 is acidic, 7 is neutral, and 7.1 to 14 is alkaline. For humans, the goal is 7.4.

What causes pH to get out of whack? The food we eat, for one thing. As pointed out in a 2012 article published in the *Journal of Environmental and Public Health*, just about everything you put in your body has its own pH. Imbalance occurs more frequently in people with diets that are too high in acid-producing foods (low on the scale). The worst offenders include:

- Cakes, pastries, commercial baked goods
- Dairy products (cheese, ice cream, milk shakes, and so forth)
- White flour and foods containing it
- Juice (commercial)
- Meats (including fish, chicken, and turkey)
- Pasta
- Boxed cereals
- Sodas, including diet sodas
- Sugar, all forms

If your diet is acidic—because you eat a lot of the foods I listed above—your body may be siphoning off vital minerals, particularly calcium from your bones, to neutralize the acid, according to the same article I mentioned above. A largely acidic diet also tends to be high in toxins, which leads to fatigue, lifeless skin and hair, and hormonal imbalances.

An alkaline diet has a number of positives, as noted by the *Journal of Environmental and Public Health* article. For example:

- An alkaline diet is high in fruits and vegetables, which improves the ratio of potassium to sodium in the body (more potassium and less sodium). When this ratio leans toward more sodium, the body becomes too acidic. An improved potassium-to-sodium ratio benefits bone heath, preserves curvy and fat-burning muscle, normalizes blood pressure, and prevents stroke.
- An alkaline diet naturally increases growth hormone (which stimulates growth, cell reproduction and regeneration). The net effect is protection against heart disease, less aging, better body composition (more muscle and less fat) and weight control, and improved memory and thinking skills.
- An alkaline diet increases the magnesium in your cells. Magnesium is an amazing mineral, essential to our bones, muscles, nerves, and immune system. An optimal supply of magnesium in the body may protect against high blood pressure, heart disease, and diabetes.

The ideal diet should include 70 to 80 percent alkaline-forming foods and 20 to 30 percent acid-forming foods. But the typical Western diet contains something like 80 to 90 percent acid-forming foods, thanks to the fact that most of us eat too much processed garbage and far too few fresh fruits and veggies.

Any diet you'll hear about from me includes the proper balance of alkaline to acidic foods, along with plenty of water to flush acid from the system, promote healthy weight loss, and improve digestion. The best foods are most fresh fruits and vegetables and certain nuts and whole grains, such as almonds and quinoa. As soon as you move toward a plant-based diet, indulging in lots of vegetables, a prudent amount of fruit, and other plant foods, your body will quickly and happily go alkaline.

4. THE CLEANSE FIGHTS CRAVINGS

Food cravings are a major culprit in weight gain, but you can control them better if you understand the physiology behind them. A desire for chocolate, for example, doesn't mean you need a Hershey's bar; it often means you are low on magnesium, which can be taken in a pill or by eating a handful of nuts or seeds. When you want potato chips, your body might be saying it needs something crunchy or higher in fat. A healthy alternative is to reach for some raw unsalted almonds, which help satisfy the need to crunch and are high in healthy fat.

Look, I get it—sometimes almonds or a magnesium supplement just won't cut it. The goal is to nourish your body in order to prevent the cravings in the first place. When you're still getting them, we must look at the *why*, and often it's an emotional thing. You're bored, sad, lonely, or depressed, and junk food can smother those feelings—but only temporarily.

Next time you have a craving, instead of reaching for the first thing you see, ask yourself if you are actually hungry. Try drinking a glass of water; you could be mistaking dehydration for hunger. When we're angry or stressed, we typically want to chew crunchy things. Raw cacao nibs, raw nuts, or a crisp apple are great options. Feeling down and want to reach for the ice cream? Swap it out for some banana ice cream with a dash of honey and vanilla extract. For this nutrient-dense and simple recipe, all you need is 1 or 2 frozen bananas. Blend them up until smooth with a little honey and a dash of vanilla extract, and either eat it like that or pop it back in the freezer for a texture more like ice cream. The new trend for this is called 'nana ice cream, and I have a few delicious recipes on my website to try post-cleanse.

If you are menstruating and craving chocolate, a handful of nuts and seeds may do the trick, but if not, it's okay to pick up some raw or

70-percent-plus dark chocolate. Once you begin to eat different things during a craving, you'll find you no longer want the food that leaves you feeling heavy or bloated.

I've put together a chart of common cravings, what each means you are missing, and a healthy replacement.

WHEN YOU CRAVE . . .	YOUR BODY REALLY WANTS . . .	TRY EATING THIS INSTEAD . . .
A burger	Fat	Sliced avocado
Sweets	Chromium	Fresh fruit or sweet potatoes
Chocolate	Magnesium	Nuts, seeds, legumes, or fresh fruit
Salty foods	Calcium, chloride, potassium, vitamin E	Unsalted nuts (such as almonds), fresh fruits, or vegetables
Carbs (such as bread or pasta)	Nitrogen, vitamin C, chromium	Almonds, citrus fruit, broccoli, grapes, or beans
Red meat	Iron, zinc, and amino acids	Organic chicken and turkey, wild-caught salmon; green vegetables, like watercress, kale, and broccoli; mushrooms; and nuts

Junk-food cravings are not natural. We weren't even born with them. They're learned traits. The good news is, we can unlearn them. This detox will help kick cravings to the curb by giving your body the essential nutrients it needs to thrive.

So, there they are: the guiding principles behind my detox. It doesn't require a radical overhaul of your behavior, just a shift toward better choices. And when you make that shift, you'll make a big difference in your health.

Next up: the foods you get to eat. Let your cleansing adventure begin!

CHAPTER 3

WHAT
TO EAT
FOODS THAT CLEANSE
AND PEEL OFF POUNDS

Thank you for giving me a plan for more energy, less bloat, and help with my sugar cravings. I'm on day five and I feel *good*! Not hungry, puffy, or sluggish. My skin is clearer and my cravings are gone. I'll be adding these recipes to my weekly meals and detoxing to get back on track as needed.

—Jennifer

Unless you try it, you can't imagine how wonderfully simple and straight-forward cleansing can be. You can find these foods at any grocery store, and the meals are delicious and easy to prepare. The portions are ample and filling, so you won't feel hungry at all. The next five days will zip by.

You'll be eating five meals daily, made up of delicious, nourishing ingredients designed expressly for detoxification. I've supplied a list of approved foods for you in this chapter; anything not on the list is off-limits for the next five days. You'll notice that certain foods that you might think are healthy (like bananas, sweet potatoes, and vegan protein powders) are missing, and this will be explained. Here's a rundown of exactly what you'll eat, and why.

CLEANSING PROTEINS

The word "protein" originates from the Greek language and means "of prime importance." I love this description. Among its many responsibilities, protein helps to make enzymes, hormones, antibodies, and about a zillion other things that your body needs to function optimally. Our bodies generally don't turn to protein as an energy source unless we have no other options. We burn carbohydrates first, then fats, and finally, in less-than-ideal circumstances, our muscles, which are made up of protein.

In terms of hunger, protein is more satisfying than the other macronutrients and requires more energy to break down and assimilate. When you digest protein, its component amino acids are released into your intestinal tract. These amino acids then pass into your bloodstream, and your body reassembles them into muscle and other body tissues for repair and regeneration. And where carbs can spike your blood sugar and insulin, protein does not.

The U.S. Centers for Disease Control recommends 50 grams of protein daily, which you'll easily get as long as you eat the beans, nuts, seeds, grains, vegetables, and fruits that I recommend. Don't panic! Plant protein is as effective as animal protein for losing and managing weight, building and preserving muscle, and making the stuff our bodies need for good health. Just look at the leg of a horse (a plant-eater) and you'll be reassured that plant proteins build sleek, lean muscle, and plenty of it.

And just so you know: this cleanse is not high-protein, low-carb. Those diets tend to be too low in fiber, and thus may increase the risk of bowel problems and colon cancer. Plus, high-protein, low-carb diets are typically loaded with saturated fat, a risk factor for heart disease. And so many of the low-carb food products on the market are nothing more than processed food loaded with chemicals our bodies don't need.

You'll be getting your protein from:

Almonds

- Are high in protein and healthy fats, which our bodies need to thrive.
- Are loaded with fiber, with four times as much as cashews, ounce for ounce.
- Help control your weight.
- Create satiety (fullness).
- Are high in bone-building calcium—more than any other nut.
- Are packed with magnesium, a mineral that calms the nervous system, regulates the digestive tract, relieves stress, and boosts energy levels.

Black Beans

- Offer the highest levels of protein, fiber, phytochemicals, and the lowest amount of carbs among all beans, making them the perfect vegetable protein for detoxing.
- Have high concentrations of flavonoids, a detox phytochemical associated with lower rates of heart disease and cancer, as well as with anti-aging.
- Are the only food on the planet that has a protein-to-fiber ratio of 1:1, not only satisfying your body's needs to repair muscle but promoting digestion, too.
- Are deliciously meaty-tasting.

Chia Seeds (optional)

- Contain twice the protein of other seeds or grains, eight times more omega-3s than salmon, and twice the potassium of bananas.
- Are high in fiber, which helps sweep toxins from the intestinal tract for detoxing.
- Help trim belly fat.

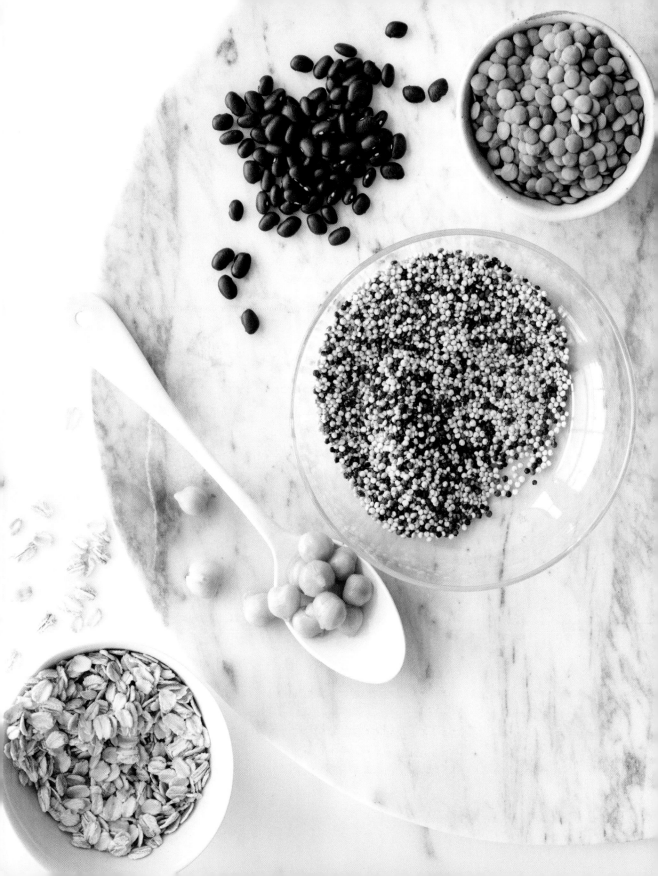

- Are filling, so you're less likely to get ravenous and grab fattening snacks later in the day. When soaked in water or other liquids, chia seeds swell up, which is exactly what happens in your tummy after you eat them, so they're an effective appetite suppressant, compliments of Mother Nature. Have 1 to 2 tablespoons a day; results guaranteed.

Chickpeas

- Help control your weight.
- Provide soluble and insoluble fibers for digestive health and detoxification.
- Are rich in two trace minerals—manganese and molybdenum—that play a key role in producing energy.
- Provide a potent source of the B vitamins folate and B_6 (½ cup supplies more than 20 percent of our daily requirement for these nutrients).
- Have a tasty, nutty flavor.
- Are flexible in meal preparation; use them anywhere from hummus to desserts.

Eggs (optional)

- Contain amino acids that are the most digestible among all proteins.
- Help increase HDL, the heart-protective, "good" cholesterol.
- Provide a rich source of the B-complex vitamin choline, which is associated with better brain function and reduced inflammation.
- Furnish sulfur, an essential mineral that helps with everything from vitamin B absorption to liver function. Sulfur also helps produce collagen and keratin, two bodily proteins that help create and maintain shiny hair, strong nails, and glowing skin.

Flaxseeds (optional)

- Deliver fiber and protein.
- Are high in B vitamins, magnesium, and manganese, all required for proper functioning of the body.
- Are rich in antioxidants and phytochemicals for efficient detoxification.
- Are the best source of lignans, which can balance female hormones. Lignans can promote fertility, help alleviate premenopausal symptoms, and may guard against breast cancer.

Lentils

- Are an excellent source of protein; 1 cup of cooked lentils has as much protein as a 3-ounce hamburger patty, but without the high amounts of fat that can clog your arteries.
- Have been found to help control appetite and increase satiety (fullness) in research.
- Deliver B vitamins for an efficient metabolism, and are high in several minerals, including potassium, calcium, magnesium, copper, iron, and zinc.
- Have a hearty flavor, making this legume a great addition to soups, stews, salads, and side dishes.
- Are easy to cook because they require no pre-soaking (unlike other legumes) and cook very quickly.
- Are less likely to produce gas, compared to other legumes.

OTHER NUTS AND SEEDS

Pick two out of this list: for example, Brazil nuts and pumpkin seeds; Brazil nuts and sunflower seeds; or pumpkin seeds and sunflower seeds.

Brazil Nuts

- Are one of the best food sources of the antioxidant mineral selenium, which is involved in metabolism and detoxification.
- Are high in fiber, which can keep you full and enables weight control when eaten in moderation.
- Represent an excellent source of monounsaturated fatty acids that help lower LDL (bad cholesterol) and increase HDL (good cholesterol).

Pumpkin Seeds

- Are high in fiber, protein, healthy fats, and many beneficial minerals, including magnesium and zinc.
- Help with muscle contraction, and since the heart is a muscle, promote a healthy heart rhythm.

Sunflower Seeds

- Are high in fiber and protein.
- Represent an excellent source of vitamin E, the body's primary fat-soluble antioxidant.
- Are rich in the mineral selenium, which is a potent detoxifier.
- Provide vitamin B_1 and the amino acid tryptophan, as well as the mineral magnesium, all of which help stabilize mood.

Tofu, Edamame, and Tempeh

- Help regulate healthy cell growth and cholesterol levels.
- Are high in protein and fiber.
- Are low in unhealthy fats.
- Offer a better alternative to meat protein, which can contain antibiotics, synthetic hormones, preservatives, and excess sodium.
- May lower the risk of breast cancer.

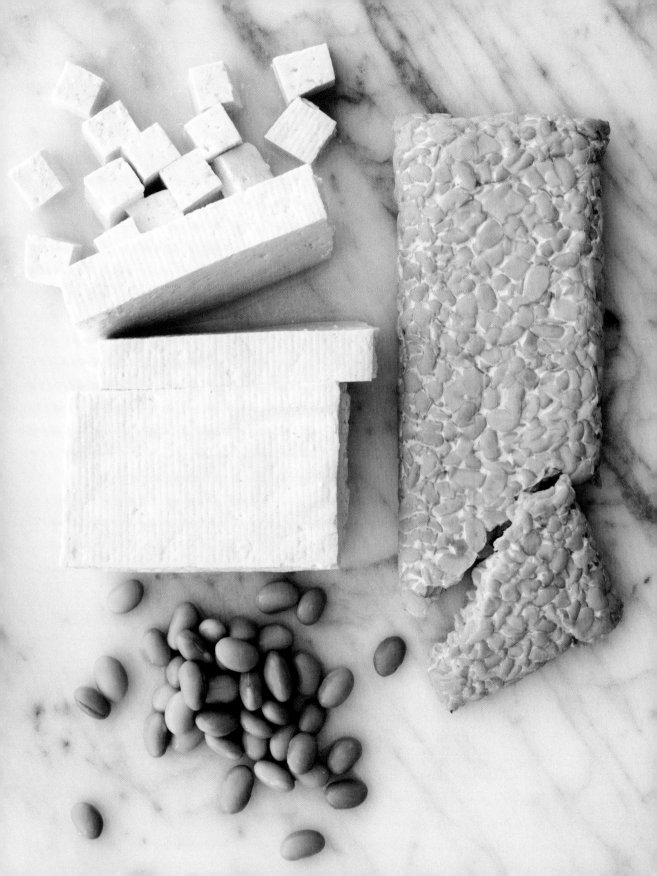

To recap, here are the proteins you'll eat on the cleanse:

- Black beans
- Chia seeds (optional)
- Chickpeas
- Eggs (optional)
- Flaxseeds (optional)
- Lentils
- Other nuts and seeds
- Tofu, edamame, or tempeh

 Note from Nikki: The Truth About Soy

Soy might just be the perfect food—in moderation, of course. It supplies fiber and important nutrients such as protein, B vitamins, calcium, and omega-3 fats. A nutritional powerhouse, soy can reduce the odds of cancer, osteoporosis, diabetes, and especially heart disease. After reviewing twenty-seven clinical trials, the Food and Drug Administration (FDA) approved the daily consumption of 25 grams of soy for lowering cholesterol levels and the risk of heart disease.

You may have heard that soy contributes to the risk of cancer. Some studies say it puts too much estrogen into your body, and others say it doesn't. So what's the real story? Once the FDA put its stamp of approval on soy, food manufacturers rushed to put it in everything. As a result, we now have soy protein concentrates, isolates, and textured soy proteins in many baked goods and processed foods like cereals, drinks, energy bars, soy meat and burgers, smoothie powders, and supplements. That's right: soy has become a processed food!

These unnatural versions of soy have hiked our consumption to dangerous levels, raising the risk of cancer and thyroid problems. In sum: it is the processed, extracted, and concentrated forms of soy that cause problems, not whole soy foods.

I feel that it's not in your best interest to be deprived of soy's benefits. Avoid isolated supplements and processed varieties, but whole unprocessed soy is healthful in moderate portions. It's best fermented, in the form of tempeh. Fermentation improves its digestibility and enhances assimilation of zinc, calcium, and magnesium.

I recommend purchasing soy products from health food stores. Be sure to look at the label to make sure it isn't loaded with unpronounceable ingredients, as well as being genetically modified (GMO) free. There's no need to be eating soy products at every meal, however. A small dash in your coffee (if nut milk isn't available) or tempeh at dinner is fine. One soy latte, tofu for lunch, and tempeh for dinner each day will become overkill for your body.

Also, if you don't like the taste of soy, skip it! It won't affect the results you'll achieve from the cleanse. I've offered some alternatives to make sure you're still getting all the protein you need.

CLEANSING VEGETABLES

These foods are the most important part of my plan, because they supply an abundance of natural detoxifiers. Cruciferous vegetables, such as cauliflower, cabbage, and broccoli, help your liver rid the body of chemicals, drug residues, and pollutants. So does spinach—a champion detoxifier among the leafy greens. Every vegetable on the list is full of antioxidants that help keep your body on guard against disease. What's more, they're packed with fiber for better digestion and weight control.

You'll be eating a huge variety of colorful and tasty vegetables, each with distinct detoxing properties. Here they are:

Beets

- Are high in fiber.
- Supply phytonutrients called betalains, which lend antioxidant, anti-inflammatory, and detoxification support to the body, particularly the liver.

- Are rich in fat-fighting vitamin C.
- Are high in red pigments called betalains that may protect against cancer.

Bell Peppers

- Are available in red, yellow, green, and orange; on the detox you'll be eating all except the green.
- Are high in vitamin C, a substance that fights both free radicals and fat, helps you to detox more effectively, and prevents various cancers and diseases.
- Supply beta-carotene, which lavishes the body with antioxidant and detoxifying benefits.
- Are a good source of vitamin E, which keeps skin and hair looking youthful.

Broccoli

- Enhances your body's ability to detoxify after exposure to food and environmental toxins, thanks to the phytochemical sulforaphane.
- Contains double the vitamin C of an orange and almost as much calcium as whole milk (with a better rate of absorption).
- Is a rich source of a flavonoid called kaempferol, which has been shown to lessen the impact of allergens in the body.

Cabbage (Purple)

- Supplies plenty of vitamins A, C, and K and folate, as well as the minerals calcium, magnesium, and potassium, making purple cabbage a well-balanced vegetable.
- Is high in glucosinolates, which destroy carcinogenic substances and hinder the growth and spread of cancer cells.

Carrots

- Are rich in vitamins A, C, and K, potassium, and B vitamins.
- Are high in fiber.
- Provide beta-carotene and alpha-carotene, powerful antioxidants that are important for detoxification.
- Are known to slow down aging and improve eyesight, and can help prevent heart disease, due to its rich nutrient profile.

Cauliflower

- Is high in glucosinolates that activate detoxification enzymes.
- Provides fiber for digestive health.
- Is rich in several anti-cancer phytochemicals like sulforaphane and plant sterols such as indole-3-carbinol.
- Is an excellent source of vitamin C and various B vitamins.

Cucumbers

- Are rich in acid-reducing alkaline compounds that help cleanse the body.
- Are high in fiber (particularly the peel).
- Work as a natural diuretic to help fight bloat, thanks to their water, potassium, and low sodium content. These qualities also help control weight gain and high blood pressure. The water content is hydrating as well.
- Reduce heartburn, flush out toxins, and aid in digestion.

Garlic and Onions

- Are rich in selenium and sulfur, both of which help flush out toxic substances that we're exposed to every day.
- Are high in vitamin C.
- Furnish flavonoids and phytochemicals.
- Are flavorful additions to many recipes.

Mushrooms

- Have been shown in studies to improve liver function, enhance the immune system, and stimulate the body's natural cancer-fighting ability.
- Are the only plant source of vitamin D, which helps with weight control and prevents many diseases.
- Are high in B vitamins, required for an efficient metabolism.
- Have a meaty flavor that enriches any dish.

Radishes

- Are a natural cleansing agent; they help to break down and eliminate toxins built up over time and enhance the activity of several liver enzymes that are part of the body's natural detoxification channels.
- Are high in powerful phytochemicals that lend this veggie its bright red outer color and protect against cancer and heart disease.
- Are high in water content and can help keep your body hydrated and your skin looking fresh and healthy.

Spinach

- Is a rich plant source of iron, required to help your body efficiently use energy.
- Is one of the best sources of dietary magnesium, required for energy metabolism; normal muscle, nerve function, and heart rhythm; a healthy immune system; and normal blood pressure.
- Contains fat-related substances called glycoglycerolipids, which appear to help protect the lining of the digestive tract from damage.
- Is considered a skin detoxifier due to its many vitamins and minerals, bringing relief from dry, itchy skin and leading to a more radiant complexion.

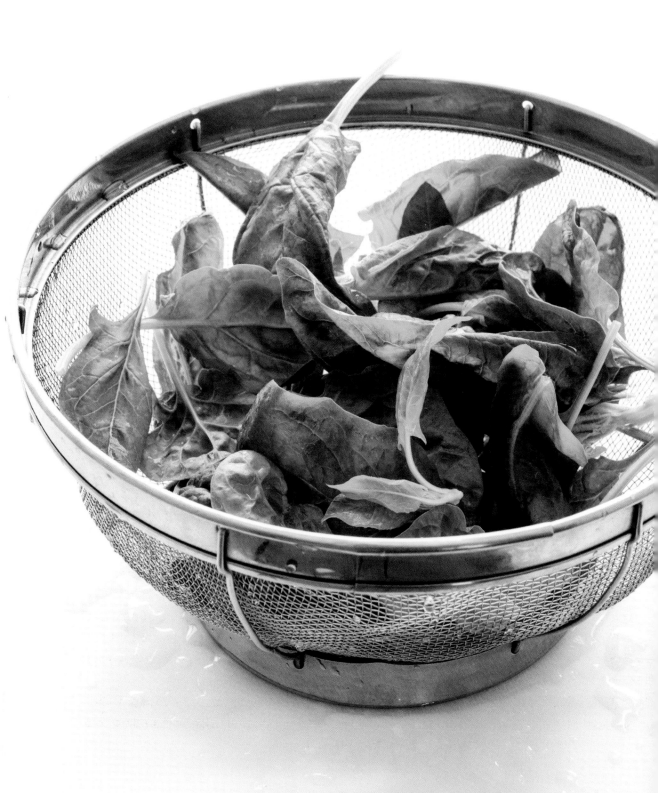

Tomatoes

- Are rich in lycopene, which provides the red color in tomatoes. Lycopene is a powerful antioxidant with cancer-fighting properties. It also helps to reduce LDL cholesterol, triglycerides, and total cholesterol, keeping your heart healthy and preventing a heart attack.
- Are high in antioxidants that protect your skin against harmful UV rays. So not only do they taste great, they are amazing for your skin as well.
- Supply vitamins A and C, the B vitamins, and potassium, all essential for metabolism and high-level health.

Zucchini

- Is high in antioxidants that help detoxify free radicals from the body.
- Is rich in potassium, helping to eliminate bloat and protecting the heart.
- Has alkalinizing properties.
- Delivers vitamins C, K, and B$_6$.
- Is versatile in meal preparation: stuff it, grill it, eat it raw, or slice it into "pasta."

To recap, here are the vegetables you'll eat on the cleanse:

- Beets
- Bell peppers (red, orange, and yellow)
- Broccoli
- Cabbage, purple
- Carrots
- Cauliflower
- Cucumber
- Garlic
- Mushrooms

- Onion, red
- Radishes
- Spinach
- Tomatoes
- Zucchini

CLEANSING FRUITS

Because they contain phytochemicals and antioxidants, fruits do an excellent job of removing built-up toxins. On the detox, you'll enjoy blackberries, blueberries, strawberries, raspberries, apples, and avocado (which is technically a fruit). All are low in sugar, carbohydrates, and calories, and high in antioxidants. The fiber they contain soaks up toxins from the digestive tract and sweeps them out of the body. Here are the specific benefits you'll obtain from these detoxifying fruits:

Apples

- Are high in phytonutrients that can help regulate your blood sugar.
- Curb hunger and enhance satiety (fullness).
- Are an excellent dietary source of soluble fiber, for detoxification, heart health, digestive health, and cancer protection.
- Are one of the leading dietary sources of boron, for bone health.

Avocado

- Is a great source of fiber, potassium, vitamins E and K, and B vitamins.
- Supplies healthy fats that help to keep you full and satiated and support healthy digestion. When you consume fat, your brain receives a signal to turn off your appetite.

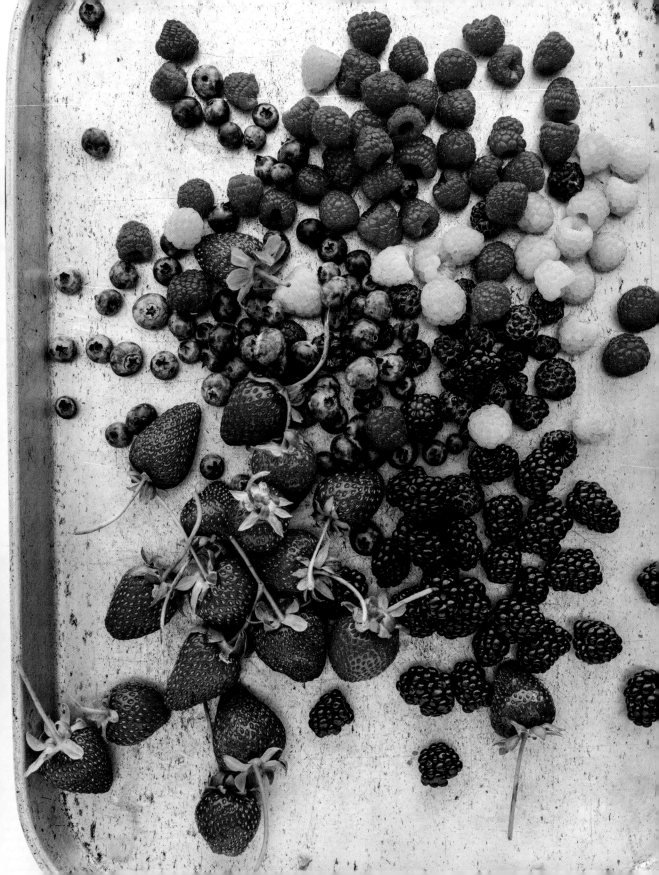

- Can be used in an array of recipes, from salad dressings to desserts (after the cleanse).

Blackberries

- Are rich in antioxidants that have proved beneficial to protect damage of cells against free radicals.
- Are high in vitamin C, which improves skin health and helps control weight.
- Provide fiber, which reduces the surge of sugar and helps the body detoxify.
- Supply a phytochemical called cyanidin-3-glucoside, which inhibits the growth and spread of cancer cells.

Blueberries

- Contain a high concentration of antioxidants.
- Are low in natural sugar.
- Help lower blood pressure, one of the leading issues related to heart attacks.
- Supply selenium, potassium, copper, zinc, manganese, anthocyanin (a phytochemical), vitamins A, C, K, and B vitamins.

Lemons and Limes

- Are a natural diuretic that gently flushes water from your system to combat bloat.
- Are high in vitamin C and other antioxidants that strengthen your immune system and help fight everything from the common cold and flu to serious illnesses.

Raspberries

- Are a highly concentrated source of phytochemicals that play a role against cancer, aging, and inflammation.

- Deliver antioxidant vitamins such as vitamin A and vitamin E.
- Supply minerals like potassium, which regulates water balance; manganese, which helps produce a key antioxidant enzyme; and copper, which is required for the manufacture of red blood cells.
- Are a good source of vitamin B_6, niacin, riboflavin, and folic acid, all of which help the body metabolize carbohydrates, protein, and fats.

Strawberries

- Are packed with vitamin C.
- Are high in fiber.
- Are low in natural sugar.
- Represent an excellent source of the trace mineral manganese.
- Supply phytochemicals called anthocyanins and ellagic acid that have benefits against cancer, aging, and inflammation and neurological diseases.

To recap, here are your go-to fruits:

- Apples
- Avocados
- Blackberries
- Blueberries
- Lemons and Limes
- Raspberries
- Strawberries

CLEANSING GRAINS

Terrified to let a carb slip through your lips? Don't be! The two grains you'll eat on the detox, oats and quinoa, will do amazing things for your waistline and overall health. Both contain protein, which is a bona fide fat-burner and tissue repairer. Most people don't think of carbohydrates as containing much protein, but these two pull double duty (of the two, quinoa has more). Plus, they'll keep you energized throughout the day so that you won't have to ply yourself with cup after cup of coffee.

Oats

- Increase satiety (fullness).
- Are high in fiber that flushes out your digestive tract.
- Are rich in minerals like manganese, selenium, magnesium, zinc, and copper.
- Are naturally gluten-free; however, oats can become contaminated with wheat, barley, or rye during the growing and/or manufacturing process. It's important to get 100 percent gluten-free oats (noted on the box) if you have celiac disease or a gluten sensitivity, but if you are not comfortable eating oats or cannot, it's fine to replace them with quinoa flakes.

Quinoa

- Contains all nine essential amino acids, making it a perfect protein for a plant-based diet.
- Is a great source of lysine, an amino acid that plays a valuable role in cellular repair.
- Is rich in the antioxidant vitamin E to help cleanse your system and give you glowing skin, hair, and nails.
- Furnishes high levels of manganese, magnesium, phosphorus, folate, copper, iron, and zinc. These essential vitamins, nutrients, and minerals help reduce blood sugar levels, keep the body healthy and strong, and keep your digestion running smoothly.
- Is gluten-free.

To recap, here are the two grains you'll eat on the cleanse:

- Oats
- Quinoa

CLEANSING HERBS

As a model, I was lucky enough to travel the globe and try foods in many different countries. I fell in love with the diverse flavors and was fascinated by how cooks at all ends of the earth could so skillfully blend fresh herbs and spices to create the most exquisite dishes—and often without any salt and sugar. Now I cook with herbs virtually every day.

Introduce yourself to basil, cilantro, and mint, and the beautiful benefits they'll give you.

Basil

- Is rich in vitamins A and C, two powerful antioxidants that help regenerate tissue for anti-aging effects, promote a healthy immune system, and protect the body from the effects of pollution.
- Provides vitamin K, essential for normal blood clotting.
- Has antibacterial properties and contains health-protecting flavonoids.

Cilantro

- Is packed with minerals such as iron, magnesium, and manganese, which promote better sleep, reduce stress in the body, and build muscle.
- Is high in antioxidants.
- Can combat lead and other heavy metal toxicity.
- Has anti-anxiety effects.

Mint

- High in antioxidants.
- Is a calming and soothing herb that has been used for thousands of years for an upset stomach.
- Helps to speed and ease digestion.
- Counters cravings for sweet foods.
- Naturally sweetens dishes without adding sugar or sweeteners.
- Has a calming and soothing effect on the body.

To recap, here are the herbs you'll include on the cleanse:

- Basil
- Cilantro
- Mint

CLEANSING SPICES

I love experimenting with spices, too. They not only perk up the flavor of any dish but also have powerful healing and detoxification powers. The five I emphasize are black pepper, cayenne pepper, cinnamon, ginger, and turmeric. Use liberally, along with fresh herbs, and you won't even miss salt or sugar.

Black Pepper

- Is used in traditional Eastern medicine for digestive disorders, including bloating, indigestion, and diarrhea.
- Contains a constituent called piperine that helps the body absorb antioxidants, vitamins, and minerals.

Cayenne Pepper

- Lends heat and spiciness.
- Is a fat-burner.
- Helps break up mucus in the body, which prevents colds and the flu.
- Promotes movement in the lymphatic system, leading to increased detoxification.
- Helps stabilize blood pressure.

Cinnamon

- Fights cravings for sweets.
- Enhances metabolism.
- Helps the body repair tissue.
- Has anti-inflammatory properties.
- Helps control blood sugar.

Ginger (optional)

- Helps treat nausea, inflammation, and diarrhea.
- Has anti-bacterial properties.
- Produces a calming action on the digestive tract.
- Has been used traditionally to relieve feelings of anxiety.
- Lends a spicy sweetness to foods. My two favorite ways to enjoy ginger are by brewing a ginger tea and adding it into smoothies.

Turmeric

- Has powerful anti-inflammatory properties.
- Contains an active ingredient called curcumin, widely used in traditional Asian medicine.
- May be helpful in treating rheumatoid arthritis, inflammatory bowel disease, dementia (including Alzheimer's disease),

**heart disease, diabetic eye problems, and cancer, according
to many studies. The common denominator of all of these
diseases is chronic inflammation, which turmeric can
alleviate.**

To recap, here are the spices you'll include on the cleanse:

- Black pepper
- Cayenne pepper
- Cinnamon
- Ginger (optional)
- Turmeric

CLEANSING WITH FLUIDS

A vital principle of any cleansing program is to drink plenty of fluids,
starting with water. The healing power of water should never be under-
estimated. It is essential to nearly every bodily process, including metabolism, digestion, absorption, circulation, and excretion. We can live
without food for five weeks, but we'll die in five days without water. It
keeps our body hydrated and restocks fluids lost through breathing and
perspiration. It facilitates bowel and urinary functions, and it flushes out
excess hormones, fats, and toxins.

Water is also a fat-burner. Your kidneys need water in order to filter
out waste products. Without enough, they turn to the liver for backup.
One of the liver's key functions is to mobilize stored fat for energy. By
taking on an overtime assignment from the kidneys, the liver can't do its
fat-burning job as well, and as a result (surprise!), you won't burn as
much fat. Drink enough water, and you'll keep your body's processes
humming along. Water can quash cravings for foods you shouldn't eat.
So if you find yourself wanting something unhealthy, reach for a glass of
water first. Dehydration can be confused with hunger, so chug away, as
long as it's that precious H_2O!

Water is also scientifically proven to reduce wrinkles, increase the

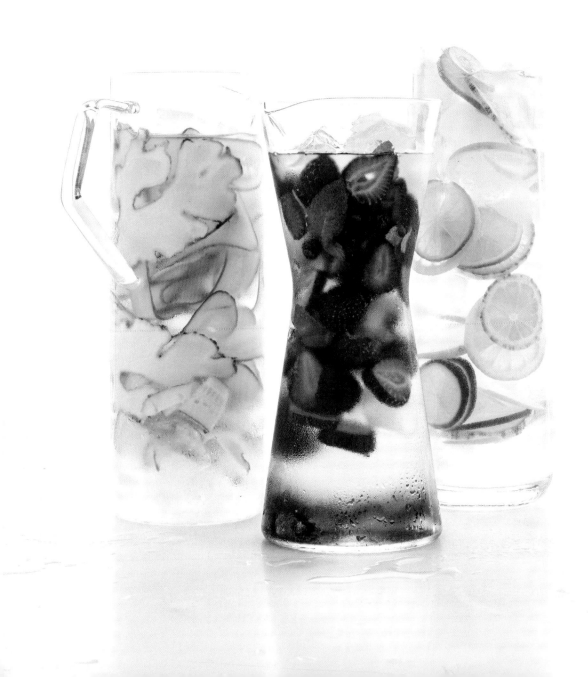

"plumped" look of your skin, and create a youthful glow. Water makes you beautiful, both inside and out.

While following the cleanse, drink 2 to 3 liters daily to enhance your results. What is the best type of water to drink? I'm not too picky here; just stay hydrated!

That said, the very best water comes in glass bottles, because you avoid any toxins found in plastic bottles. Another good option is to filter your water through a charcoal system such as Brita. Tap water is fine, too. I feel strongly that it's more important to be drinking your daily dose than to spend money on bottled waters that come with often unfounded health promises.

 Note from Nikki: How to Pimp Your Water

- Apple cider vinegar (only a dash is needed, which will aid in digestion; drink it a half hour prior to eating)
- Berries: strawberries, blueberries, blackberries, raspberries
- Cucumber
- Ginger
- Lemon, lime, and orange slices
- Mint
- Basil
- Rosemary
- Spirulina (a natural green powder that provides an energy boost), baobab (the powder of an African fruit), or chlorella

Simply chop your ingredients and add to a jug or mason jar and fill with water. Let it sit for at least 20 minutes, preferably in the fridge. The water will get infused with nutrients and flavor it for a refreshing and satisfying treat. Once you've finished your water, keep the fixings in the jar and refill it! I refill using the same ingredients for one or two days. Try to get ingredients that are in season. They tend to be cheaper, which means you won't be spending an arm and a leg for your fancy water. When a certain variety of produce is in season, stock up, freeze it, and continue to toss it in year-round.

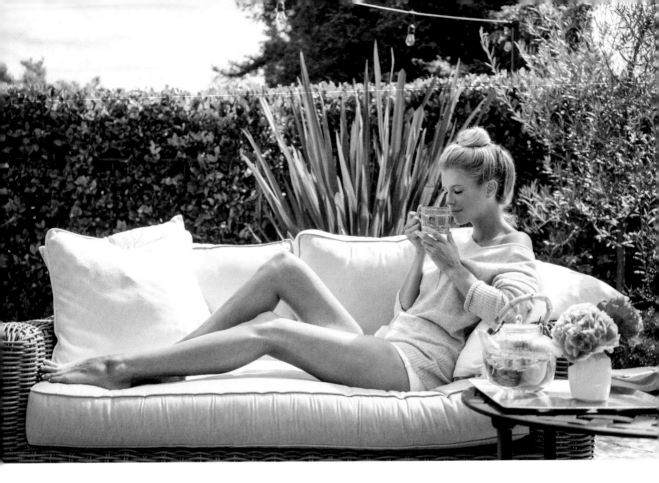

While most detoxes do not recommend caffeine, I include green tea (and matcha green tea powder) because going cold turkey is a shock for the body and extremely unpleasant. And if something is unpleasant, you're less likely to stick with it.

Luckily, green tea offers the best of both worlds. It happens to be abundant in natural chemicals called catechins, which promote fat-burning and stimulate thermogenesis, a calorie-burning process that occurs after digesting and metabolizing food. According to a study published in the *International Journal of Obesity* in 2010, green tea can increase your metabolism by as much as 4 to 5 percent. Other research tells us that green tea helps protect against heart diseases, cancer, and inflammatory bowel disease.

If you don't love green tea, worry not. Herbal teas will help you drink more water and enhance your results, too. My favorites are peppermint, which aids indigestion; fennel, to reduce bloating; and ginger, to soothe the tummy and boost immunity.

I love to try new teas, too. Each time I do the cleanse, I grab a new flavored green tea and various herbal teas, and mix and match to create my own. Try it! You'll find out what you like and what really hits the spot (especially during a craving). Drink 2 to 4 cups a day of mainly herbal tea, with 1 cup of green or matcha tea in the morning or whenever you would normally crave coffee.

There you have it—all the wonderfully delicious foods, herbs, and spices you get to enjoy for the next five days. The variety will help you break your usual routine. And the new eating habits you develop will help you keep the bloat off and lose even more weight.

To ensure that my detox is 100 percent effective for you, there are also some substances you'll want to avoid for five days. That's where we're headed next.

CHAPTER 4

GIVE YOUR BODY A BREAK
ANTI-CLEANSE FOODS

I've struggled with my weight and my horrible eating habits since I was in elementary school. At age nineteen now, I almost settled for the thought that I'd just be overweight for the rest of my life. Then I found your cleanse. I took a chance on it, and I'm so happy I did. My bloating is gone. My stomach is nearly flat. It was the best feeling the other day to step out of my car as I arrived at work, only to realize that I need a belt, because my jeans are a bit too big for me now. I've discovered so many new ways to eat deliciously and keep my body clean and happy all at once. I still have miles to go, but the cleanse has given me the motivation to carry on.

—Vanessa

The cleanse works best when you faithfully stick to the meal plan and keep yourself well hydrated. That's why, for the next five days, you're going to give your body a break from certain substances that can impede your results. By cutting out specific foods and beverages, even briefly, you'll reverse their toxic effects, rid your system of impurities, and help your body work at its full capacity.

Although I want you to focus intensely on what you *can* eat (so much goodness!), I do want you to be aware of the stuff that can interfere with detoxification. During this five-day period, don't touch:

Alcohol

- Is one of the most commonly ingested toxins.
- Is broken down into acetaldehyde, a toxin that does damage to liver cells, the brain, and muscles.
- Inhibits digestion, causes dehydration, and compromises the functioning of the central and peripheral nervous systems. The cumulative effect can be constipation, which interferes with detoxification.
- Increases calorie intake and bloat.
- Keeps you from reaching the deepest, most restful, and healing stage of sleep, known as REM (rapid eye movement), leaving you feeling tired the next day. When the body hasn't had enough sleep, it looks for energy from sugar and fat.

Artificial Sweeteners

- Are chemicals, and we're detoxing from chemicals.
- Stimulate your appetite, creating food cravings, as your body is not getting proper nutrition. They also increase carbohydrate cravings and stimulate fat storage and weight gain.
- May make you eat fewer nutritious foods, in favor of artificially flavored foods with less nutritional value.

Caffeine (with the exception of green tea) and Caffeinated Beverages

- Disrupts digestion, which is a key part of detoxing.
- Prevents your body from digesting and absorbing all those nutrients, which will be flushed out of your system, defeating the whole purpose of any detox meal.

- Can contain high amounts of sugar, fake sugars, various chemicals, or dairy, all of which we want to avoid.

Dairy Products

- Are acid- and mucus-forming; both compromise the body's immune response.
- Are among one of the most processed foods you can consume, particularly cow's milk.
- Are typically pasteurized, which destroys many vitamins and enzymes typically found in raw milk.
- May contain hormones, antibiotics, and substances from inorganic grains, fed to cows to increase milk production. The chemical residues from those processes wind up in the milk we drink (unless we buy organic milk).
- May contain toxins. According to multiple studies and reviews, if a mother cow feels distress or hears distress signals from other cows when their calves are taken away, she secretes toxins into the milk—which we then drink. Think of our own fight-or-flight mode, in which our chemicals change when we feel we are in danger (typically triggered by stress).
- May be hard to digest because of the lactose (milk sugar). If you're intolerant of lactose, you'll feel bloated and susceptible to embarrassing gas. Be very careful about the dairy you eat and drink, or don't have it at all.

Meat and Other Animal Proteins

- Can produce sluggish digestion. The human digestive system, versatile as it is, is better suited to a plant-based diet. Compared to fruits, vegetables, and grains, animal foods move very slowly through the body. The longer meat stays in your system, the more time it has to form deadly carcinogens.
- May be riddled with antibiotics, hormones, contaminants, and other toxins.

- Tend to be high in saturated fat, which contributes to heart and artery problems.
- Are acid-forming.

Packaged Foods and Fast Foods

- Are usually laced with chemicals that can slowly poison your liver, kidneys, and other vital organs. Read the ingredient list sometime; it's likely to be full of unpronounceable additives. And if you can't pronounce it, it is definitely bad for you.
- Loaded with ridiculously high amounts of salt, sugar, fat, calories, and often chemicals to give them a longer shelf life (particularly fast foods).
- May claim to be "healthy." Beware: even "healthy" fast food may be full of chemicals. Your typical sandwich bun is a good example; it can contain more than twenty ingredients, including GMO (genetically modified organisms) ingredients, and enough sugar and calories to exceed what your body needs in a week.

Protein Powders

- Are highly processed—including vegan powders—and therefore not natural.
- May contain up to thirty ingredients, particularly whey powders.
- Lead you to believe they will help you gain muscle with no negative side effects. Building muscle is a function of how intensely you train and how well you feed your body with natural foods, namely real protein, either from lean animal sources or plant sources, and good-quality carbohydrates. Remember, the cleanse is based on real food, not anything that you'd find in a package or canister.

Salt

- Causes water retention, which leads to bloating.
- Is less effective for seasoning foods than fresh herbs and

spices, which will aid in digestion as well as give ample amounts of flavor to your meals.

- Can clog your arteries because of its mineral content, just like rust builds up in a pipe. This can lead to high blood pressure, stroke, coronary heart disease, obesity, and kidney stones, among other negative side effects.

Sodas and Diet Sodas

- Increase the risk of obesity. Harvard researchers have calculated that each regular soda you drink increases your risk of obesity 1.6 times.
- Contain numerous chemicals.
- Can be high in caffeine, depending on the product.
- Contain the equivalent of up to 10 teaspoons sugar (one can of regular soda).
- Contribute to serious diseases, mainly because they contain high-fructose corn syrup, which has been associated with increased risk of metabolic syndrome, potentially leading to diabetes and heart disease.
- Contain phosphoric acid, which can block calcium absorption and lead to osteoporosis, cavities, and bone softening. Phosphoric acid also interacts adversely with stomach acid; this reaction can interfere with digestion, block nutrient absorption, and impede detoxification.
- May contain aspartame (diet sodas), which has been linked to seizures, multiple sclerosis, brain tumors, diabetes, and emotional disorders. Aspartame turns into methanol (an alcohol used in racing car fuel) at warm temperatures, and methanol breaks down into formaldehyde and formic acid, both harmful chemicals.
- Destroys teeth by dissolving tooth enamel and causing plaque to build up, leading to cavities and gum disease.

Sugar (all forms, including honey, coconut sugar, date sugar, agave, and stevia)

- Is highly addictive, even more so than cocaine or heroin.
- Contains no essential nutrients.
- Can overload your liver (particularly added sugars, and especially high-fructose corn syrup).
- Contributes to diabetes, heart disease, and possibly cancer.
- Feeds bad bacteria in your gut, increasing the likelihood of skin irritations, fatigue, digestive problems, mood swings, bloating, headaches, among other nasty conditions.
- Causes tooth decay (regular sodas).

Read Labels for These Chemicals

The following food additives are suspect when it comes to good health, and will also interfere with detoxification. Be sure to check food labels and avoid anything containing them.

ADDITIVE	HEALTH CONCERNS
Artificial colorings	Blue 1, Blue 2, Citrus Red 2, Green 3, Orange B, Red 3, Red 40, Yellow 5, and Yellow 6. Found in candy, soda pop, gelatin-based desserts, and many other processed foods, artificial colorings can trigger allergies.
BHA and BHT	Preservatives put in foods to stop fats and oils from turning rancid. Scientific studies indicate that they cause cancer in lab animals. Both are found primarily in packaged cereals, chewing gum, snack foods, and some vegetable oils.
Potassium bromate	Used mainly in commercially produced bread, this is a dough conditioner that makes dough more spongy and soft. It is also a bleaching agent. Various studies show that it may cause kidney tumors in rats. You'll find it in white flour and in white bread and rolls.
Propyl gallate	A preservative to prevent spoilage in foods containing fats and oils. Numerous animal studies show that it may trigger tumor formation. Found in vegetable oil, meat products, potato sticks, chicken soup base, and chewing gum.
Sodium nitrite and sodium nitrate	Found in bacon, lunch meats, corned beef, and virtually any smoked, cured, or processed meats in order to stop bacterial growth. Also, cancer-causing substances called nitrosamines may form in the body after ingestion.
Sulfites	Trigger breathing difficulties, rashes, abdominal upset—even, rarely, death. Found primarily in dried fruit, wine, and processed, packaged potatoes.
TBHQ (tert-butylhydroquinone)	A preservative used in some vegetable oils, snack foods, fast foods, packaged cereals, and other fat-containing foods. It has been found to increase the incidence of tumors in rats. TBHQ is similar to butane, used as a lighter fluid.

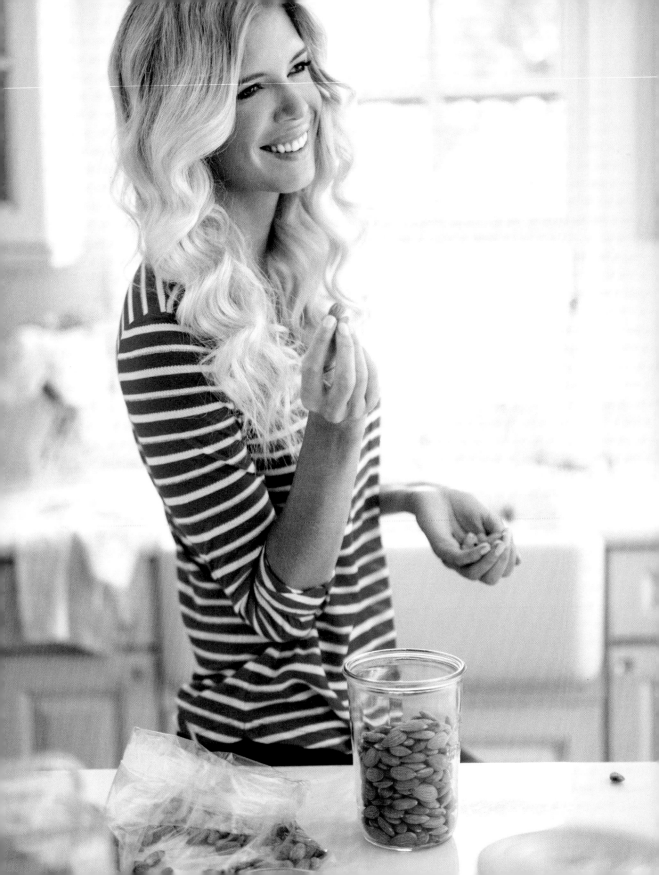

BUT WHERE ARE THE BANANAS?

I get asked all the time why certain healthy foods, such as bananas, sweet potatoes, and winter squash, are off-limits during the five days of the cleanse. Simply put, they're high in starches, low in protein, and not as high in fiber as the foods chosen for the detox. I absolutely recommend them long-term as part of a healthy diet—and as soon as you finish the cleanse, you may be craving a delicious banana. But for now, stick with the dos and don'ts listed previously.

Now, I'm not saying that you can never eat those foods ever again, or that you should forever stick with my recommendations. It's my job to explain to you how to get healthy and achieve the body you want. In life, as in diet, balance and moderation are critical to getting and maintaining results, so if you want to order a diet soda at lunch someday, I'm not here to stop you. All I'm asking is that for five days you leave a few things on the shelf—and I know it ain't easy (remember, I grew up eating mac and cheese and Lunchables). But if you do, expect to see a lighter, leaner body that will make you think twice about the dishes you normally go for.

Remember, all the luscious foods you *do* get to eat have been chosen very specifically. Trust me: You'll see amazing results when you follow the plan as it's written.

CHAPTER 5

THE PRE-TOX

I went from 129 pounds to 122 pounds. I ate whole foods the entire time. I sleep solidly now, having suffered from sleep problems and fatigue my entire life. I will hold on to these basics for the rest of my life.

—Jessica

Okay, now you are mentally ready to detox . . . so what's next?

It's time to get in gear with what I call the "pre-tox"—the preparation phase of the 5-Day Real Food Detox. Detoxing does not mean just changing the food you eat. It means tossing the junk from your pantry, stocking your kitchen with the right foods, and getting your mind in gear. The pre-tox is critical to the entire process. If you take the time, it'll lead to success, dedication, and, perhaps most important, confidence that your efforts will pay off.

DECIDE WHEN TO START

Some days are better than others to start the plan. I've found that it's best to begin on the Sunday or Monday of a quiet week at work, or a week without a demanding schedule. That'll take you right up to the next weekend, when you're slimmer, lighter, and more energetic. You may even be able to fit into a smaller dress size by Saturday.

If you're a woman, I don't recommend starting while you're on your period. Your appetite and cravings might be surging out of control, and if you're feeling moody, you won't be psychologically ready. So wait until your period passes, and aim for a day when you feel physically and emotionally at your best.

You can also follow the detox if you're pregnant, but check with your physician first. According to Helen Phandis, the dietician I worked with in developing the cleanse, "You and your baby will get most of the vitamins and minerals you need, but you should also take a daily pregnancy multivitamin and a mineral supplement containing 10 micrograms of vitamin D and 400 micrograms of folic acid."

Of course, if you're recovering from a serious illness or having medical treatment for any condition, please postpone the detox until your doctor gives you the go-ahead.

But don't put it off for too long. Why? Because every day counts. The sooner you start, the closer you'll get to the life you deserve.

EASE INTO THE CLEANSE

Some of you may be eager to start immediately, and that's great! Jump right into it and start seeing results right away. It's also okay, though, if you want to go slow, depending on how unhealthy your eating habits have been over the past few months. Look over these four statements and check any that apply to you:

- You drink more than one cup of coffee daily.
- You have milk, cheese, yogurt, or any other dairy products once a day.
- You eat fast food or pre-packaged meals at least once a day.
- You dine out more than three times a week, including lunch.

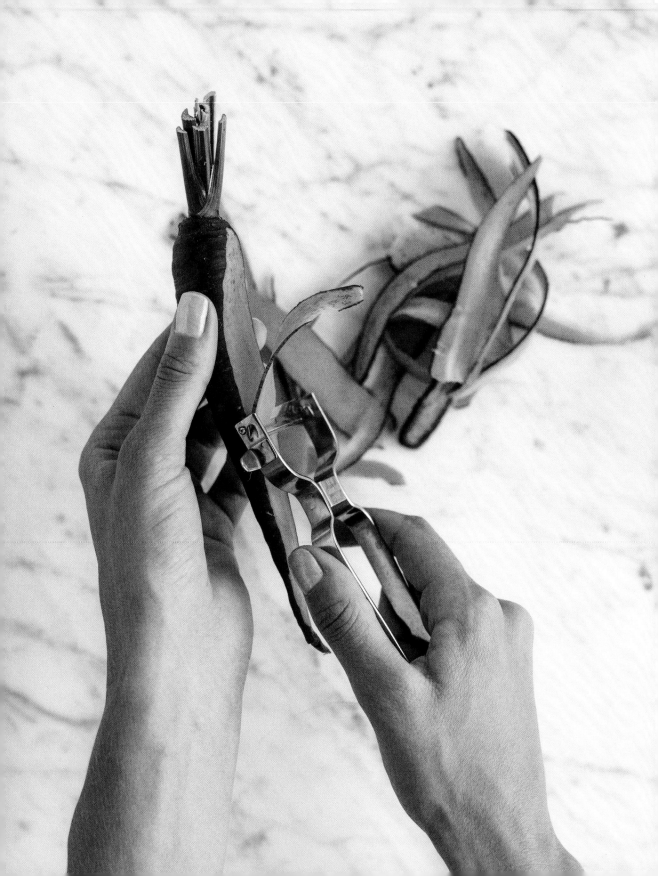

If one or more of these statements describe you, then you should start slowly, so that you don't feel overwhelmed or go cold turkey on everything you enjoy. I've had people telling me that they couldn't get through even one day without caving, or they had such bad headaches that they couldn't focus on work. Easing in will prevent these issues from cropping up.

Make small changes to your eating habits for a few days first. Baby steps will set you up for even better results and make it easier to complete the cleanse successfully. Here are some mostly-painless options:

For the next five to seven days, choose one of the four habits that you acknowledged above, and make that your starting point. For example, if you're a habitual coffee drinker, cut down to one cup a day, or if you drink only one cup a day, swap it out for green tea.

Then, if you're feeling good, cut something else out, such as dairy, soda, diet soda, afternoon candy snacks, processed food, or fast food. Abstain from anything that is pre-packaged, such as chips, cookies, or sandwiches, and don't eat anything that has more than five ingredients listed. Start eating at least one piece of fruit or a salad a day. Another way to prep is to have my Detox Smoothie each day (see page 122) as a supplement to your regular meals.

If eating out is your downfall, cut back; designate Friday or Saturday as restaurant night so it's more of a special occasion. It'll also get you in the good habit of preparing your own meals and paying closer attention to what goes into your body.

If you commit to all of this, your taste buds will gradually adjust, and you'll stop craving salt, sugar, coffee, and alcohol. You'll begin to desire natural foods instead, and feel mentally and physically prepared for five days of beautiful, cleansing foods.

CLEAN OUT YOUR KITCHEN

Set up your surroundings for success. This means clearing out any tempting foods from your pantry and refrigerator. Why give your body a chance to re-pollute itself? At the end of each day, you'll be happy that you didn't cave in to any junk—because you removed all of it!

Below is a suggested list of foods to consider tossing. This is optional; I don't want you to throw away everything you like in life. However, I do want you to be conscious about trigger foods that may be too hard to resist when you have a craving or feel tired and hungry after an exhausting day. I find it's best to not have these foods in my house at all, but I do realize sometimes that's not realistic, especially if you have a family or live in a shared apartment. So if you can, give these foods away, trash them, or put them in a double-tied trash bag and hide them in a closet. Put your favorite candy out of sight, and you put it out of mind. There! Your willpower just got stronger.

Consider ditching, hiding, or donating (during the detox):

- Alcohol—beer, wine, liquor, and cocktail mixes
- Baked goods, including breads
- Candy
- Cheese
- Chips
- Coffee
- Cookies
- Crackers
- Fried foods
- Frozen meals
- Juice, commercial
- Ice cream and other frozen desserts
- Milk and other dairy products
- Soda, including diet sodas
- Sugar
- Salad dressings, ketchup, and soy sauce

Read labels and remove all foods containing:

- Additives you can't pronounce
- Aspartame and other artificial sweeteners
- Brown sugar
- Corn syrup
- Dextrose
- High-fructose corn syrup
- Honey
- Hydrogenated oils
- Maltodextrin
- MSG
- Raw sugar
- White flour
- White sugar

GO SHOPPING

You now have plenty of room for your healthy detoxification foods. It's time to head to the grocery store, or to your local farmers market for the freshest food available. To help you, I've prepared a shopping list (see page 77).

When you get to the store or market, try to buy mostly organically grown foods, which are not treated with pesticides or other chemicals. It's a smart move to purchase from sources that are chemical-free—local farmers and ranchers who use sustainable production methods, for example. Fortunately, even many regular grocery stores now have aisles stocked with organic foods. Ask the produce department which day of the week fresh fruit and vegetables are delivered. Fresh is always best.

Eating organic is important not only to successful detoxing but also to healthy living. A 2014 study reported in the *British Journal of Nutrition* revealed that compared to conventionally grown foods, organic plant foods have higher levels of antioxidants and phytochemicals, all of which help your body properly detox. The study also pointed out that pesticide residues were four times higher in the conventional crops than in the organic produce. Why ingest more chemicals than you need to? Organic produce is our best bet.

Is it pricier? Yes, but those prices are coming down as we consumers demand organic. I used to be one of those people who'd pinch every penny when it came to grocery shopping because for many years I earned very little. My epiphany came when I realized how much of our food is sprayed with pesticides, genetically engineered, and transported long distances, losing nutrient value on the way. Why was I even considering buying apples that had been treated with chemicals, flown in from Europe, and trucked all the way across the United States? Now I try to go to farmers markets and purchase organic from my local shops. Depending on the season, it's not always that much more expensive, and it tastes so much better. I'd rather cut back in other areas of my life to be healthy and chemical-free.

Scout out Asian and Indian markets, where things like big bags of almonds, seaweed paper, and cans of chickpeas and black beans are typically much less expensive. (Make sure the beans are in BPA-free cans.) Many large grocery stores now have international sections, where they sell nuts, seeds, grains, and other items for a fraction of the cost of the other aisles. You can buy staples such as beans, nuts, seeds, and grains in bulk from markets that allow you to fill your own bags, which also saves money. Lastly, if you cannot find a certain item in your local store, search online, because there are many websites now dedicated to shipping tofu, nuts, and even fresh food. Sites such as Amazon sell huge bags of almonds and other seeds at much cheaper prices than elsewhere. You can also order online from community farmers and co-ops. Get the most bang for your buck.

You may still feel that you don't have the cash to buy all your groceries organic, and I get it. If you can manage to swing one or two organic items off my shopping list, that is a great start. Get to know the Environmental Working Group's Dirty Dozen list of the most toxic conventionally grown fruits and vegetables—the ones you should prioritize buying organic—as well as their Clean 15, the produce that contains little to no chemicals, whether or not it's organic. Check it out at www.ewg.org.

As for the cleanse, what will your grocery bill look like? I spend around $80 for all five days—and this includes buying organic. I already have things like olive oil, cinnamon, cayenne, and tahini (sesame seed butter) in my pantry, though, so you can expect the bill to be around $100 if you have to start from scratch. This might seem like a lot of money to spend in one go; however, the grains, olive oil, and seasonings will last long after the cleanse is over.

Think about it: $100 is for five meals a day for five days. That breaks down to $4 a meal (again, if you have to buy *all* the ingredients), which is cheaper than your typical cup of coffee! Plus, you'll have leftovers—that means further savings. One final tip: try not to shop on an empty stomach, or you may end up purchasing food you don't need and probably shouldn't eat. Stick to the list. Once you're done I give you full permission to head back to the store and buy whatever else you want, but for these five days, bring home only what's needed.

The Shopping List

Proteins

One 16-ounce package of raw almonds

Pick two: 6.3-ounce package of Brazil nuts, raw pumpkin seeds, or raw
sunflower seeds

One 15-ounce can chickpeas*

One 15-ounce can black beans*

One 16-ounce package dried green lentils

One 16-ounce package white or red quinoa

One 2-pound bag rolled oats

One 14-ounce package firm tofu

6 eggs**

*I personally buy these organic and canned (BPA-free); however, it is
more cost-effective to buy dried legumes, beans, and chickpeas. You'll just
have to remember to rinse and soak them overnight.

**Optional, but necessary if you make the Love Pancakes or Eggs-cellent
Breakfast and you are not replacing with chia seeds.

Produce

One 16-ounce bag or box of raw spinach

3 avocados

2 portobello mushrooms

1 cucumber

1 zucchini

1 head of broccoli

1 head of cauliflower

1 package of cherry tomatoes or 3 large tomatoes

One 1-pound bag of carrots (or 4 large carrots)

1 small head of purple cabbage

2 red bell peppers

1 yellow pepper

1 large beet or 3 small ones

1 small bunch of radishes

1 small red onion

1 head of garlic

Fruits

6 lemons

3 limes

4 cartons or bags of berries (fresh or frozen): blueberries, raspberries, blackberries, and strawberries*

3 to 4 apples

* I recommend getting whatever is in season and fresh to save money; otherwise, pick two to three cartons, such as blueberries and strawberries, or blackberries and raspberries, and so forth. Frozen unsweetened berries are fine, too, and cost less than fresh berries.

Fresh Herbs

1 bunch basil

1 bunch cilantro

1 bunch mint

Spices

Black pepper

Cayenne pepper

Cinnamon

Turmeric

Other suggested spices: Chinese five-spice powder, cumin, paprika, and ground ginger

Extras

Small bottle of extra-virgin olive oil

One 16-ounce jar of tahini

Balsamic vinegar

Apple cider vinegar

1 pack of nori seaweed papers

Green tea

Mint tea

Fennel tea

If you're a guy doing the cleanse, or your guy will be doing the cleanse with you, you'll have to purchase more food, so consider at least doubling up on what I've listed.

THE PREP

I suggest you do a little food prep the day before starting the cleanse so you have everything you need at your fingertips. Some suggestions:

- Prepare the Spinach & Chickpea Hummus (page 133) ahead of time and store in a bowl in your refrigerator. I personally like to pre-portion the hummus into five small containers, which are easy to grab each day.
- Cook your quinoa and lentils ahead of time, too, so that they're ready to toss into other dishes. (See my instructions on pages 129 and 137.)
- Portion out your meals. If you are short on time and make a few of the meals in one sitting, add them to five containers so you are less likely to overeat on one meal and have less on the next.
- It's best to chop veggies up right before eating them so they keep all their nutritional value, but if you know you won't have time, dice or shred them and place them in individual containers in your refrigerator.
- Make the salad dressings ahead of time and refrigerate.
- Place your smoothie ingredients for each day into a plastic bag and throw it in the freezer. That way, in the morning, you can just put the contents into your blender with water and ice, rather than taking time to measure everything.
- For convenience, I buy canned chickpeas and black beans, but I rinse them carefully. Buying beans in bulk can save money, however. If you buy the uncooked variety, soak the beans overnight. The following morning, rinse and drain them. Cook in simmering water until soft (this may take up to 3 hours). See my instructions on page 137 for preparing uncooked beans.

DETOXIFIED!

I'm a thirty-year-old married mom of three; my youngest is four months old. I love health and fitness and was on my fitness journey prior to doing the detox, but wow, has this been a huge game changer! I thought I was eating pretty clean before, but I realized I actually wasn't. I was a little over-

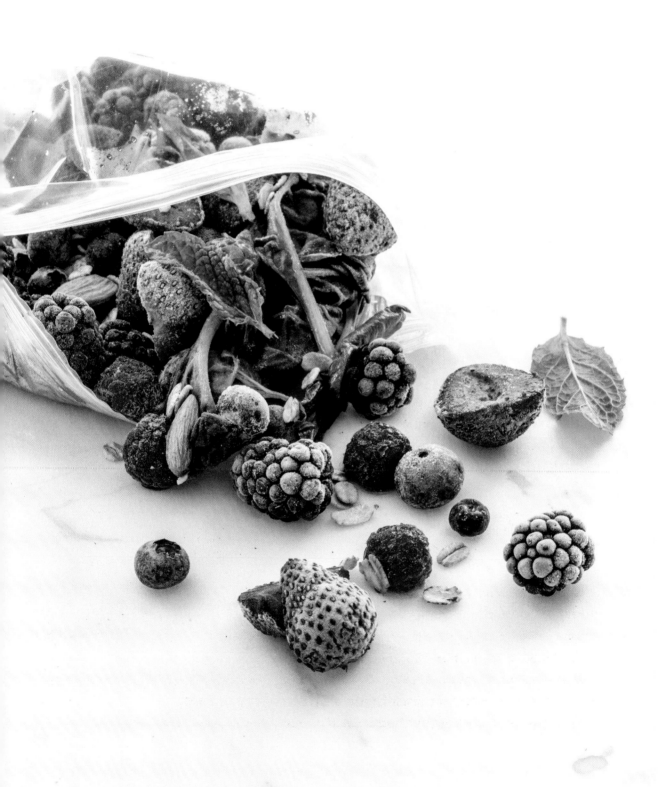

whelmed at first because I had never really prepped my entire day or week of food in advance. Nor had I ever gone without coffee, dairy, or meat. But I was committed and excited to do it. I ended up losing 7 pounds along the way!

I've taken so much from this experience, from prepping my food and incorporating a huge variety of veggies and fruit to preparing healthy snacks and meals for my husband and kids instead of the processed stuff we used to buy. Why has this changed my life so significantly? Because of the way I feel physically, emotionally, and mentally! You don't realize how much the foods we put into our bodies affect our mood, clarity, and overall well-being until you actually change your diet for a while and experience it. Which is what happened to me.

—Michelle S.

TAKE THE "BEFORE" AND "AFTER" PHOTOS

I know it can be scary to take a "before" photo, and trust me, no one likes doing it. But when you finish the detox and see how flat your stomach is, you'll be so glad you did! The "before" and "after" photos, which you should take on days one and six of the cleanse, are one of my favorite ways to see the changes that can happen, because you might not actually believe how much weight you can lose or how tight your body will feel.

Below are some tips for taking these photos, which I promise you will value come day six (this is where my modeling experience comes in handy!):

1. Be consistent. Take your photos at the same time of day, wearing the same clothing, and in the same mirror. Morning shots are best because the natural light is better, which means you'll get clearer photos.

2. Minimize the clutter. You don't have to clean your room as if the in-laws are coming, but a photo always looks best with a clean background and in a mirror that doesn't have a ton of water marks on it.

3. Learn the angles of your body. Stand in front of the mirror (with phone in hand) and figure out if you look best straight on or if you should turn 45 degrees. Does your face look better tilted to the side, or with one shoulder up toward your face and the other one down?

4. Use a photo timer app or video on your phone. This is one of my tricks. When I take a photo that's not in the mirror, I use the timer app (free) or the video on iPhone and extract a screen shot when I find a pose I like.

I know these tips might seem over the top, but trust me, once you see how much of a difference the detox makes, you'll want to share your transformation with the world! But more important, those pictures are concrete proof of your accomplishment, which can be very motivating. Even if you've never heard of Facebook, those photos will come in handy the next time you need a gentle kick in the butt.

Please remember that the cleanse will produce different results each time you do it. If you don't see what you're after the first time around, don't fret! I've done it so many times, and something new always happens; sometimes I lose more water, sometimes I get more energy, and sometimes it's harder. But through it all, taking "before" and "after" photos is one of the best things I've done to track how my body responds.

DON'T GET CAUGHT UP IN NUMBERS ON THE SCALE

I know some of you like hard data, but if you must, please only weigh yourself the days before and after the detox, when you take your photos. Don't focus on your daily weight, because it may fluctuate, discouraging you and impeding your progress. Just believe that it's working, even if you might occasionally feel bloated or constipated during the five days. The goal here is to change how you look at food and how you feel about your body, to change your habits for lifelong health.

Besides those precious selfies, other markers of progress may be a flatter tummy or looser clothes, all of which will encourage you to finish strong.

DETOX YOUR SOCIAL CALENDAR

Stay focused by not participating in any events that involve food or alcohol. Parties, bars, and restaurants are out. Some things are just too seductive when you're trying to detox, and social events are one of them. In Chapter 11, I'll give you some guidelines for making healthier choices out at restaurants and social functions once you finish. Just remember, this is only for five days, which I know you can do!

ESTABLISH THE RIGHT MINDSET

Your number one success factor will be getting your head in the right place. Success starts from within. If you're not fired up, no cleanse can help you feel better. You have to be single-minded—totally focused for the full five days. It's not about simply changing your eating; it's about changing the way you think about food and your body. This is actually easier than it might sound. There are a few simple things that I recommend prior to starting and if any roadblocks come up during the five days:

- **Visualize what's important.** Is it being able to ease into a smaller size? Feeling lighter and more energetic? Maybe it's kick-starting your weight loss? Finally getting rid of that acne that has been plaguing you? Or looking fitter at forty-five than you did at twenty-five? Whatever your goal, remembering *why* you decided to challenge yourself will keep you on track.
- **Release bad thoughts.** If you're thinking that you can't do it or that you'll fail, you'll limit your chance of success. Every time obstructive thoughts (such as "I can't stick to this") come to mind, imagine those words on a balloon that you're holding. Then see yourself releasing that balloon into the sky until it's no longer in view. This powerful visualization will help you release negative thoughts.
- **Start loving yourself—and your body.** Sit down and write out ten of your greatest assets. Are you a great friend? A good cook? A loving mom? A smart money manager? Do you have great hair? Beautiful

eyes? Strong biceps? What body parts do you really like? This list should give you a boost. If you ever feel like throwing in the towel, take it out and remind yourself why you are *worth it*. Focus on the good! Every time you find your thoughts going negative, write down something positive. It seems overly simple, but it works.

- **Use affirmations.** Repeat these silently to yourself or post them where you can see them, and think of them as a detox for your brain. Some examples:
  - *The detox is an act of love toward my body.*
  - *I can do this detox, and I'm excited about its benefits.*
  - *Every day that I detox, I am honoring my body, my health, and my life.*
  - *Today I'm becoming slimmer and fitter.*
  - *I enjoy nourishing myself with fresh, healthy meals instead of processed food.*
  - *When I eat well, I feel well, and my life is positive and joyous.*
  - *I am mindful of where my food comes from and what is in it.*
  - *Doing this detox means taking better care of myself.*
  - *My health is a precious gift. I will respect it and cherish it daily.*
  - *I will take time to enjoy the food that is nourishing my body and my life.*
  - *Just as I cleanse my body of toxins, I also cleanse negativity from my emotions and thoughts.*
- **Promise yourself a reward for completing the detox.** This could be new jeans or a sexy bathing suit for the summer, workout shoes, a massage, a mini-vacation—something spectacular that excites and motivates you. But it must not be food. In other words: no pigging out at the end of the cleanse! You're on the path toward changing your eating habits for a lifetime, and that'll just undo the great work you've already done.

Finally, whatever you want from this detox, visualize having it, accomplishing it, living it, and enjoying it. Allow yourself to feel the positive emotions attached to success—the joy, happiness, pride, and excitement from living in a healthy, vibrant body.

Are you ready? Let's cleanse!

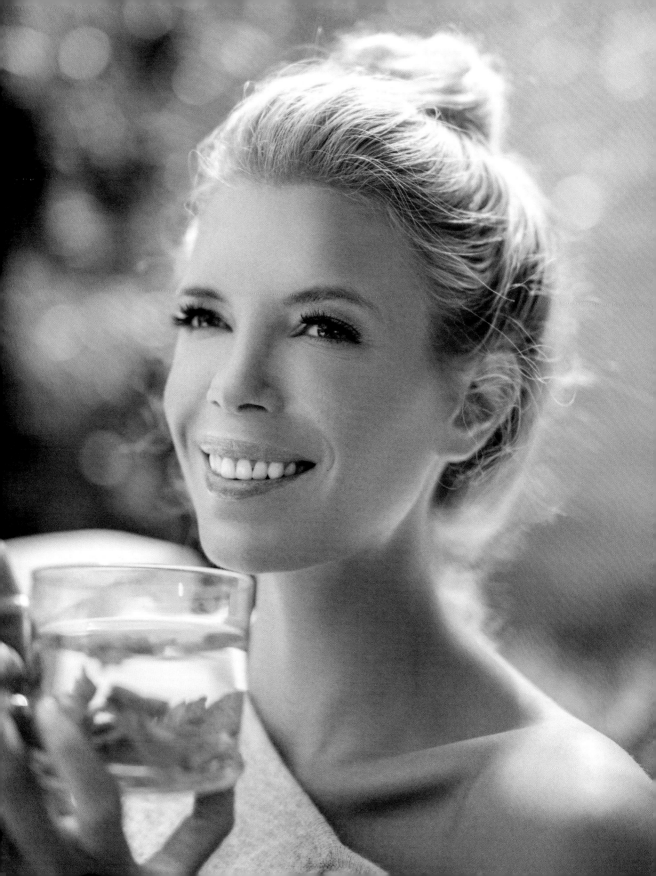

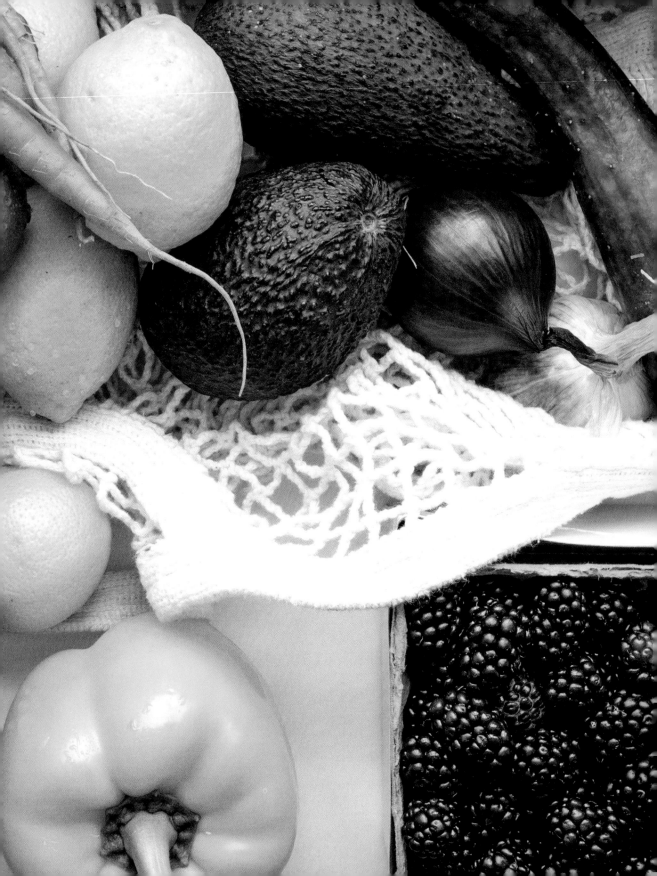

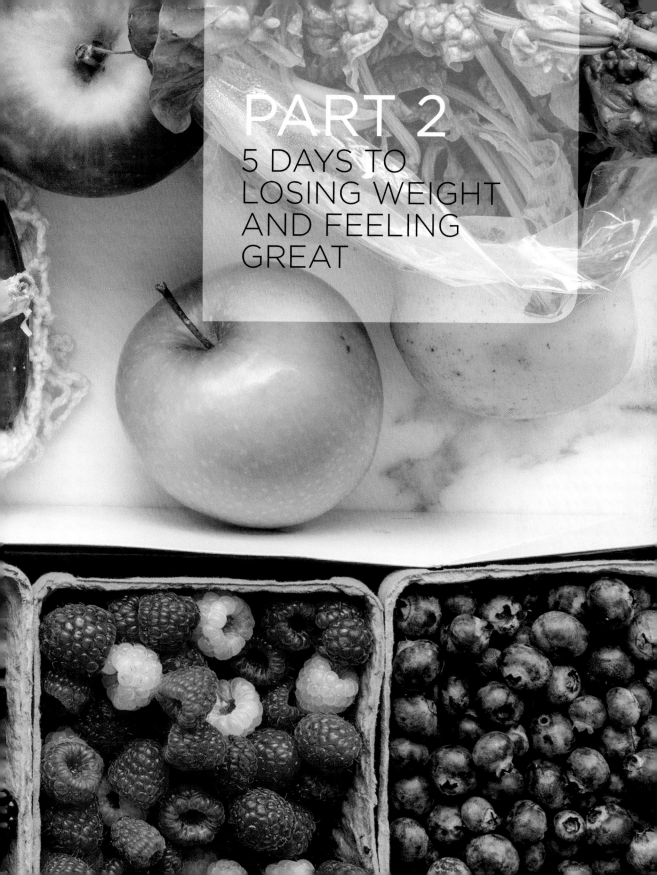

PART 2

5 DAYS TO LOSING WEIGHT AND FEELING GREAT

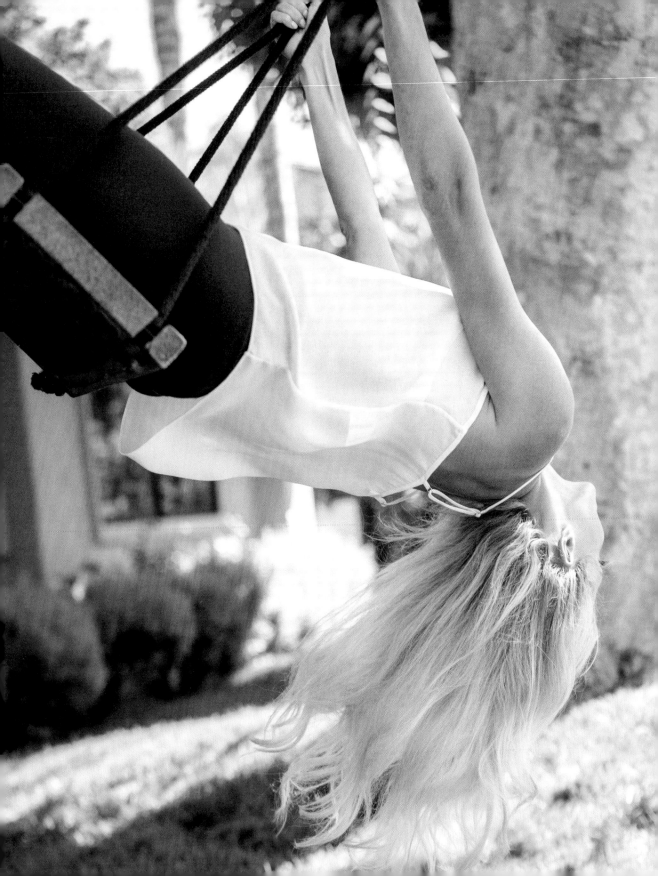

CHAPTER 6

THE 5-DAY PLAN

I've had horrible morning sickness throughout my whole pregnancy. I haven't been able to keep anything down but crackers and ginger ale. It's been so frustrating! I'm so hungry, and I thought I should do a detox because I believe in the power of fruits and veggies. And guess what—it's only the second day, but I haven't felt ill at all. I'm just so grateful, and I plan on eating this way for the rest of my pregnancy.

—Jordan

It's time to begin! Day by day, you'll witness a remarkable transformation in your body. Eating only clean, natural foods will give it a well-deserved break from salt, sugar, chemicals, and other nasty things added to what we normally eat. Expect to shed excess weight and relieve bloating. Watch your energy soar. Let me remind you that after the detox is over, you'll have glowing skin and, hopefully, a little less cellulite.

All of this in five short days!

WHEN YOU WAKE UP

As soon as you get up in the morning, sip a cup of warm lemon water. Squeeze the juice of one-half large lemon or one full small lemon into a mug of warm-to-hot water and stir. Warm lemonade:

- Stimulates your digestive system and liver—organs that are the most active in the morning. Unless you're using the toilet regularly, it's difficult to lose weight. Plus, poor digestion can block your body from getting the nutrition it needs to manage your weight.
- Increases the acidity of the digestive system, which is the one part of your body that you want to be a little acidic. An acidic digestive system helps the body absorb calcium and then store it in fat cells. The more calcium there is inside a cell, the faster the cell burns fat, as reported in a 2003 *Journal of Nutrition* article. Also, some studies have hinted that calcium keeps tabs on a hormone called calcitriol, which causes the body to produce fat and interferes with fat-burning.
- Cleanses the colon and speeds up the elimination of toxins.
- Kick-starts your metabolism.
- Provides more vitamin C than an orange. Vitamin C may well be a fat-burner, especially if you want a flat tummy. Researchers from the University of Cambridge in the United Kingdom analyzed blood levels of vitamin C and body-fat distribution in nineteen thousand men and women. They discovered that people with higher blood levels of vitamin C had less fat around their bellies. This study was published in 2005 in the *American Journal of Clinical Nutrition*.

Consider fortifying your lemon water for an extra boost. Add ⅛ teaspoon turmeric and ⅛ teaspoon cayenne pepper, along with a dash of apple cider vinegar. This upgraded version will not only reduce your cravings but also give your metabolism an extra kick, along with encouraging the detox process. I love turmeric, and you'll find it in a ton of my recipes; it's one of the best ingredients you can choose for cleansing your body quickly.

Wait twenty minutes after you've had your warm lemonade to eat breakfast.

BREAKFAST

Morning meals are a mix of foods to help give you energy and keep you full without leaving you feeling heavy. Having breakfast gives your metabolism its daily jump start so that when you eat later, your body burns calories and fats efficiently. Breakfast also keeps you from getting overly hungry later in the day. In short: skipping breakfast can actually make you gain weight! If you don't like breakfast, don't worry, because your choices are light and will help you get in the daily habit. Eating too much food at any meal is more likely to clog your system and deenergize your body.

During the next five days, you have four breakfast choices—and thus lots of variety:

- Detox Smoothie (page 122)
- Energizing Oats (page 125)
- Love Pancakes (page 126)
- Eggs-cellent Breakfast (page 129)

SNACKS

Snacking is vital to a successful cleanse. It minimizes blood sugar spikes and supplies you with ample energy in between meals. All of my snacks are simple to prepare and take with you to school or work.

You get to enjoy two snacks a day. One of these is a homemade spinach hummus with a combination of carrot, cucumber, or tomato slices, which provides carbohydrates, fats, protein, and extra vegetables to keep you full. It's absolutely delicious, and if you're anything like me, it will be hard to stick to only one portion a day! Remember, it can be made ahead of time and refrigerated. Divide the batch into five smaller containers for portion control and to make it easy to grab and go.

Other options are an apple with sunflower or pumpkin seeds, or berries with Brazil nuts. I recommend that you eat your fruit snack later in the day to fight the typical afternoon slump in which you might eat something sugary for a pick-me-up. Fruit is nature's candy—and a great late-in-the-day choice.

A word of caution, though: do not have your second snack late at night. If you didn't have time for both snacks or didn't need both, end your day with dinner. Eating at night can prevent you from wanting breakfast the following morning, and it interferes with sleep and your body's restorative processes. Late-night noshing can weigh down the body and mind. One last piece about snacking—if you are seriously not hungry, don't force yourself to eat. Just make sure you're not skipping snacks for the sake of reducing calories, as this will hinder the detox. Start listening to your body and its hunger signals.

LUNCH

You'll get to choose from five lunch options. Yes, you heard that correctly! Five delicious lunches, a different one every day if you wish. To ensure maximum gains from the plan, lunch is mostly raw. Why?

1. Raw foods take longer to digest; eating them midday gives your body plenty of time to break down and absorb their nutrients.

2. Fresh, raw food gives you enzymes necessary for elimination, letting your body detox, heal, and fight off disease or inflammation more effectively.

3. Natural, uncooked foods are free of processed waste such as trans fats, artificial additives, and added sugars. They're high in detoxing compounds such as phytochemicals and antioxidants, vitamins like folate and vitamin A, and minerals such as potassium and magnesium. A study published in the *Journal of Nutrition* found that eating raw foods can lower total cholesterol and blood triglycerides, decreasing the chances of heart disease, the number one killer of U.S. adults.

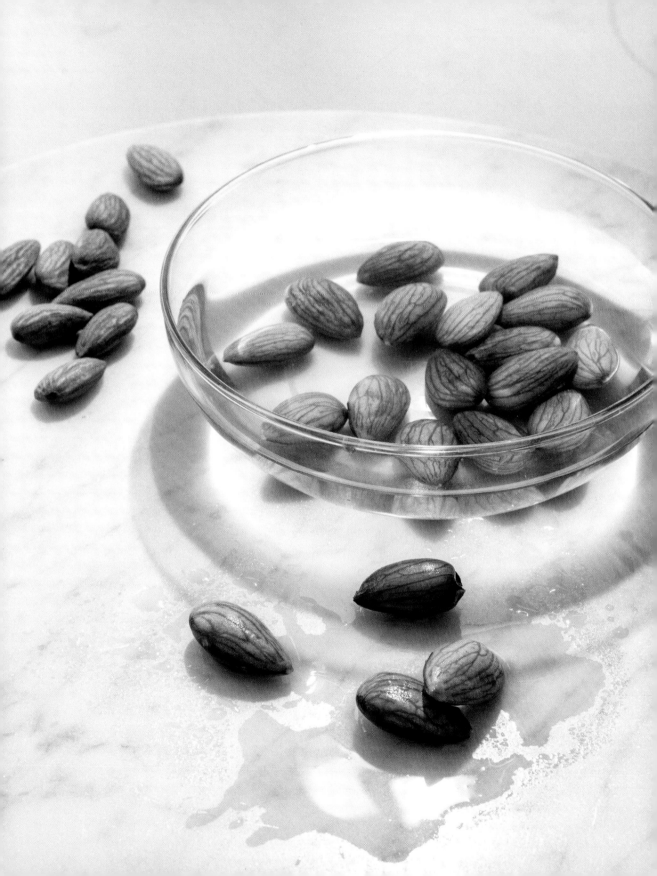

4. My favorite reason to enjoy raw foods on occasion: they're colorful and delightfully crunchy.

The lunches are all different but easy to prepare, and very filling. They are:

- Superfood Salad (page 134)
- Spiralized Noodles (page 139)
- Colorful Crunch Salad (page 140)
- Sushi Rolls (page 143)
- Taste the Rainbow Salad (page 147)

DINNER

My plan is designed to maximize your digestion for more efficient detoxification. So at dinner, your meals are cooked. Remember that, unlike raw foods, cooked food is easier for your body to break down later in the day and early evening—and thus easier on your digestive system and less likely to cause bloating. I also find it comforting and satisfying at the end of the day. Cooked foods also offer these distinct nutritional benefits:

1. Some phytochemicals, such as the carotenoids found in tomatoes and carrots, are not as easily absorbed from raw foods. Cooking these foods breaks down cell walls to unleash these nutrients. Stewed tomatoes, for example, give you more lycopene (a phytochemical) than raw tomatoes, and cooked carrots offer more beta-carotene than raw.

2. The minerals magnesium, calcium, iron, and zinc, which are naturally present in many foods, are more available to the body when those foods are cooked.

3. Heating food makes it more digestible, allowing for better absorption of much-needed nutrients.

4. Cooking vegetables makes the fiber more soluble, for more efficient regulation of blood sugar and digestion.

5. Cooking destroys many harmful bacteria.

All of the dinners will meet your daily nutrient requirements for protein, carbohydrates, fats, vitamins, and minerals.

Your options are:

- Sensational Stir-Fry with Cauliflower Mash (page 148)
- Roasted Red Pepper (page 153)
- Taco Bowl (page 154)
- Black Bean Burgers with Slaw (page 157)
- Cleansing Cabbage Bowl (page 158)

THE 5-DAY REAL FOOD DETOX

Here is your eating plan and schedule for the next five days. Mindful eating is key, so enjoy your meals in a calm environment. Sit down when you eat, and go slow, chewing every bite completely before swallowing. Sip the Detox Smoothie over a period of twenty minutes to fill you up and reduce blood sugar spikes (which can sap your energy and leave you feeling hungry in no time).

Your Five-Day Plan

	DAY 1	DAY 2	DAY 3	DAY 4	DAY 5
UPON ARISING	Lemon water	Lemon water	Lemon water	Lemon water	Lemon water
BREAKFAST	Oats or Smoothie	Love Pancakes or Smoothie	Eggs-cellent Breakfast or Oats	Oats or Smoothie	Smoothie or Eggs-cellent Breakfast
SNACK 1	Hummus with Carrots	Hummus with Cucumber	Hummus with Tomatoes	Hummus with Cucumber	Hummus with Carrots

LUNCH	Superfood Salad	Spiralized Noodles	Colorful Crunch Salad	Sushi Rolls	Taste the Rainbow Salad
SNACK 2	Apple with Sunflower or Pumpkin Seeds	Berries with Brazil Nuts	Apple with Sunflower or Pumpkin Seeds	Berries with Brazil Nuts	Apple with Sunflower or Pumpkin Seeds
DINNER	Sensational Stir-Fry with Cauliflower Mash	Roasted Red Pepper	Taco Bowl	Black Bean Burgers with Slaw	Cleansing Cabbage Bowl

EXTRA SUPPORT FOR THE DETOX: USING SUPERFOOD POWDERS

When I embarked on my clean-eating journey a few years ago, I had no idea what a superfood powder was. It seemed like another gimmick to get me to purchase expensive things that I didn't really need. Nonetheless, I thought I'd give it a try (hey, I'd tried every other fad diet out there—why not?).

I remember opening my first packet of spirulina (a nutritional green algae) and nearly keeling over from the grassy smell. It was only after I began mixing it with lemon water and smoothies that I adjusted to the taste. But I noticed something else: I started feeling even *more* amazing than I had with the dietary changes alone. These superfood powders— with fun names like maca, baobab, and chlorella—were doing something to my body that I didn't really understand, so I began researching their benefits.

Here's the lowdown. Superfood powders—concentrated, powdered versions of nutrient-dense foods such as exotic roots or berries or green algae—have been around since ancient times. The Egyptians, Incas, and

Aztecs all used them to fuel their bodies when going out for long days to hunt and forage. The body digests and absorbs them much more rapidly than multivitamin pills, so you reap the benefits quickly. When superfood powders are taken with a healthy diet, you'll have more energy, clearer skin, and a more efficient digestive system.

Here's my advice on when and how to supplement with superfood powders, whether detoxing or not.

For greater energy: Add 1 teaspoon maca to your oatmeal or smoothie. A member of the radish family that has been cultivated for more than three thousand years in South America, maca helps the body adapt to change and stress, which is why it's referred to as an "adaptogen." It's also a great vegan source of vitamin B$_{12}$; minerals such as iodine, iron, manganese, and zinc; and protein. Studies have shown maca to increase energy, physical stamina, and endurance (and it's also thought to enhance sex drive!).

For greater hydration: Add 1 teaspoon baobab to your water and sip throughout the day. Baobab is a powder made from the African superfruit of the same name. Its strong mineral-electrolyte profile helps maintain proper water balance of your cells; it has five times more of the electrolyte potassium than bananas. It also contains six times more vitamin C than oranges, which boosts collagen and hyaluronic acid production in the skin, making it radiant.

For extra detoxing: Take 1 teaspoon chlorella daily. Chlorella is a single-cell, freshwater green alga. It boosts immunity activation, heals and regenerates tissues (including skin), and detoxes heavy metals and pesticides from your system. A 2008 study published in the *Journal of Medicinal Food* found that taken daily it helped reduce body fat, total cholesterol, and high levels of blood glucose. Chlorella may just be the perfect nutritional remedy against toxins.

For post-workout recovery: Add 1 teaspoon spirulina to a smoothie. Spirulina contains 60 to 70 percent protein. In fact, its protein is four times more absorbable than the protein in beef! Taken after a workout, spirulina helps the body recover quickly and reduces muscle pain. Spirulina is one of the most nutritious superfoods on earth, good for everyday use as well. It's loaded with omega-3s; B vitamins; the antioxidant vitamin C; the fat-soluble vitamins D and E; and potassium, iron, calcium, and zinc.

While superfood powders might sound like that "magic pill" you've been waiting for to help you detox, cleanse, and lose weight, they should only be taken as a supplement to a healthy diet. If you have to choose between spending money on organic food (or even conventionally grown but clean food) or superfood powders, I will always say buy the food. Like taking a multivitamin, superfood powders aren't going to drastically change your health, but they can give you a nutritional boost.

HANDLING POSSIBLE SYMPTOMS

Some people have no negative symptoms for the entire detox. Others do, especially during the first couple of days. Keep in mind that it's perfectly normal to experience fatigue, headaches, hunger, irritability, bloating, or nausea; these are simply signs that your body is shedding waste and toxins. Don't feel discouraged! See it as a positive sign that your body is being transformed from the inside out. Any side effects should pass after two to three days. Here are some guidelines on how to handle them in the meantime.

Fatigue

The detox is probably a major change from your normal diet. Therefore, in the early stages, you might feel a little weak and tired. On the other hand, you may feel newly energized, due to an increased intake of vitamins and minerals your body doesn't normally get.

If you feel tired, make sure you're eating all the food in the suggested portions. Make sure, too, that you're drinking enough water, since dehydration can make you lethargic. You may require more sleep than normal. If you're feeling run-down, go to bed at least a half hour earlier, or sleep in a little later the next morning. Let yourself rest so that your body can heal and replenish itself. I always find that when I'm craving coffee during the detox, it's because I haven't had enough water or food. Having a piece of fruit or noshing on a salad is one of the best ways to increase your energy without resorting to a caffeine bump.

Headaches

Headaches are common in the first twenty-four hours. This is usually because you're withdrawing from caffeine, the most widely used drug in the world and the only drug that's added to foods. You're missing your daily dose, and the headache is a form of physical rebellion.

Cutting out sugar can also trigger headaches, even flu-like symptoms in some people. Overeating sugar shares some of the characteristics of more destructive addictions. When you detox, you're eliminating a drug-like substance; it's normal to experience withdrawal.

Drinking plenty of water and having regular bowel movements can relieve these headaches. If you find you are still getting them during the detox, be sure that you are drinking some green tea, which provides a gentler form of caffeine for the body.

Still having headaches? You may need to take medication as directed, but only as a last resort. Please remember that detoxing can be tough for some, but powering through the negative side effects can make you feel better. A headache is never fun, but try to think about why you might be getting them in the first place. If it's a caffeine habit, then skipping your coffee and ibuprofen will help to relieve them in the future.

Diarrhea and Constipation

It's actually pretty common for people to get constipated during the first two days on my detox, because they suddenly increase fiber intake to levels that their body is unaccustomed to. This is another reason it's so vitally important to drink two to three liters of water a day. If you don't use the toilet within the first two days, I recommend taking an over-the-counter magnesium powder, which can help promote bowel movements. If this still doesn't work, senna tea is a natural alternative to harsh laxatives. You may also experience diarrhea, which sometimes occurs with a change in diet. If it is severe or prolonged (lasting for a couple of days), consult your doctor to rule out any medical problems. But don't worry too much. Either side effect will be temporary, as your gut adjusts. Again, make sure to drink the recommended amount of water to make up for any fluid lost.

Bloat

Because you'll be upping your fiber intake—which draws water into the gut—you may feel bloated. Paradoxically, you'll want to make sure you're drinking a lot of water—8 to 10 glasses a day, or 2 to 3 liters—to keep food moving through your system and to reduce gas. Our guts are very adaptable, and in a few days you'll find that any bloating or gas will subside. By day four, you'll wake up with more energy and a perfectly flat, beach-ready tummy.

Hunger

You shouldn't feel overly hungry or deprived, because you're eating so much filling food (unlike on liquid-only detoxes). But if you get hungry at any time, simply boost your intake of vegetables, cooked or raw. Also, make sure you're drinking enough water, since hunger is often a sign of dehydration.

I've found that when I start getting cravings for foods that are not a part of the cleanse, it's because I have gone too long in between meals. Simply put, if you try to skip meals, alter how you make them (such as cutting out fruits or the beans because they have carbs), or decrease portion sizes, it will likely backfire and lead to bingeing.

Irritability

Cutting out caffeine or sugar may make you anxious, irritable, or moody. To relax, I recommend the following breathing meditation because it clears toxic emotions and helps you calm down. All you need to do is close your eyes (if you can remember the words—it may take some practice) and on each inhale and exhale, silently say the next word to yourself. When taking the breath in, really fill your whole body, then release, allowing everything out.

Inhale: think or say "love."
Exhale: think or say "hate."
Inhale: think or say "strength."
Exhale: think or say "weakness."
Inhale: think or say "happiness."
Exhale: think or say "grief."
Inhale: think or say "bliss."
Exhale: think or say "sorrow."
Inhale: think or say "satisfaction."
Exhale: think or say "disappointment."

I suggest that you do the detox five days out of every month. That way, you can continue to rid your body of toxins that might have built up again from your diet, lifestyle, or the environment. Unfortunately, we're all still subject to environmental toxins, so cleansing once a month can protect you and keep you from plateauing with your weight loss.

CHAPTER 7

THE GUY-TOX
CALLING ALL MEN

Just an update to let you know that since I did your detox, I have stayed pointing in the right direction, eating healthy and training three times a week. I even signed up for a marathon! It was just the positive kick-start I needed. So thank you for your positivity and direction.

—James

This chapter is for men—but not for men only. Wives, sisters, moms, and girlfriends—you're welcome to read it, too, especially if you want the man in your life to benefit from the cleanse, or do it with you.

So, guys: you've probably never thought much about detoxing. It sounds too intense, or you're worried you'll essentially starve for five days. Or maybe you're actually a little curious as to what the buzz is all about. Will you see results? Can you still build muscle? Will you still feel manly? With my plan, the short answers are yes, yes, and yes. In fact, the benefits to men in particular are numerous. I'm going to dive into some hard-fact science to show you that detoxing is not only safe but a *great* idea.

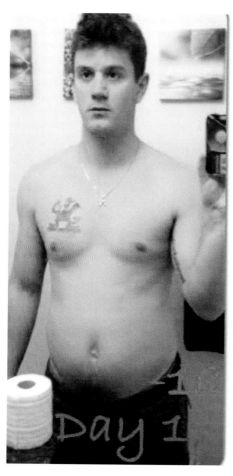
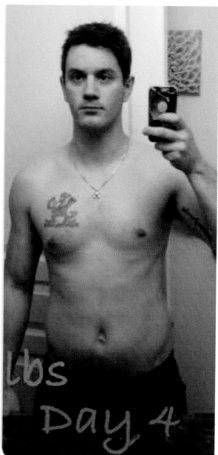

lbs
Day 1   Day 4

YOU MAY LOSE MORE THAN THE TYPICAL 5 POUNDS IN 5 DAYS

Men's and women's bodies are different (that might be the most "duh" line you've ever read!), and men lose weight faster than women do. I've seen men lose up to 13 pounds (sometimes more) in five days and uncover a high degree of ripped definition. Not only do men lose weight more easily than women, they also tend to keep it off longer, according to research published in the *American Journal of Men's Health* in 2015, in which the men studied maintained a loss of 10 pounds or more over one year but the women did not. Those guys achieved success by increasing their exercise and eating fewer bad fats, whereas the women joined commercial weight-loss groups, took prescription diet pills, and went on fad diets (clearly none of that worked well, particularly for maintenance!).

Why the big difference?

First, men generally are more muscle-bound than women, and those muscles burn lots of calories because they are metabolically so active. More muscle means burning more fat. Each pound of muscle can incinerate around 50 calories a day. That means by having even five pounds of muscle on your body, you can be burning an extra 250 calories a day! And that's without even going to the gym or watching what you eat.

A side note for the ladies: Pay attention to what I just said. Muscle is denser than fat, which will create that toned and tight look many of us strive for. The correct diet, combined with lifting weights or doing exercises with your own body weight, instead of only cardio, will increase your metabolism, burn more fat, and help you get that body you want!

Second, while men generally have less body fat than women to begin with and can lose it more quickly, the kind of fat you guys carry is something to pay a little more attention to.

You see, there are two different types of body fat: subcutaneous fat and visceral abdominal fat. Both act differently in the body. Subcutaneous fat is distributed throughout the body but is found mostly in the hips, thighs, and buttocks. As the name suggests, it lies right underneath your skin. It's the fat that jiggles when we walk or spills over when we squeeze into jeans. It's also the hardest and most stubborn to take off. But don't worry. You can fight it with high-fiber foods such as fruits and vegetables. By helping blast waste from your body, these foods rid your body of toxic obesogens that can keep you fat.

Visceral abdominal fat is just a complicated name for a bulging gut. While subcutaneous fat is mostly a cosmetic bummer, an excess of visceral fat is downright dangerous. It is linked to cardiovascular disease, type 2 diabetes, Alzheimer's disease, and other very serious illnesses. An analysis published in the *Journal of the American College of Cardiology* scrutinized data from more than 15,900 people with heart disease and concluded that those with too much visceral fat—even with a normal body weight—had twice the risk of premature death. Visceral fat is very scary news.

Guys, unfortunately you tend to have higher levels of this fat. But the good news is that it's easier to lose, particularly with the correct diet and exercise. Do some regular high-intensity workout training, decrease the bad foods in your diet, and increase the good stuff, and you will lower your risk of heart disease in no time.

Eating a lot of soluble fiber helps rid the body of visceral fat, too. Soluble fiber attracts water, forms a gel in the stomach, and helps you feel full. A five-year study of 1,114 subjects, published in 2011 in the online journal *Obesity*, found that eating more soluble fiber daily from fruits, nuts, and legumes decreased the accumulation of visceral fat in subjects by 37 percent. My cleanse provides just what you need in the form of apples, beans and other legumes, broccoli, cabbage, carrots, nuts, and green leafy vegetables.

DETOXIFIED!

I did the detox with my dad (who is quite overweight) last week, and we were so pleased with the results. Dad lost almost 16 pounds in about nine days (he continued the detox because he liked the food so much). And I lost 4½ pounds. The cleanse was so much easier than what I thought it was going to be, and it improved my sleeping as well!

—Ruby M.

YOU CAN BUILD MUSCLE MORE EFFECTIVELY

I know the big question on your mind is: Will I sacrifice muscle if I detox?

No—in fact, quite the opposite. If you want to optimize your metabolism and sustain muscle growth—and I know you do—your body requires a clean internal environment. I can't stress this point enough.

Think about it this way: You've finally bought that sports car you've been dreaming about since you were a kid. This is your *baby*. Would you put dirty, unleaded 87-octane fuel in it when you know that it can only run properly on 91-octane premium? No, you wouldn't; that would reduce performance and decrease its life span. Your body works the same way.

As I mentioned earlier, the liver is the chief organ of detoxification, but it is also involved in reactions that directly impact the growth of muscle tissue. Your immune system plays a role here, too; a healthy immune system supports the repair and growth that take place after your workouts. When you cleanse, you reduce the associated toxic burden on your liver and immune system. Consequently, both systems can direct more of the body's energy and resources toward the repair of exercise-induced muscle damage, and support more effective delivery of nutrients to tissues for better muscle growth.

Here, you'll eat a ton of fiber-rich plant foods. The fiber keeps food and waste moving efficiently through your gastrointestinal tract, purging toxins from your system so that you can recover more quickly from your workouts. Better recovery leads to more muscle growth.

Once you start eating more vegetables, your digestive system will start to improve, and you'll begin to take off extra pounds more easily. (Constipation impedes weight loss. So while you might not care if you're getting backed up, it may be preventing you from seeing results.) Couple this benefit with the fact that you'll be getting off bloat-inducing sodium. *More fiber plus less sodium equals visible muscle definition in only five days.*

Drinking 13 cups of water daily also plays a vital role in your efforts to burn fat and maintain lean mass. Water is one of the most powerful muscle-building nutrients ever. I simply can't overhype it. Water dilutes, dissolves, and helps push out toxins that could otherwise constrain your immune function, recovery, and muscle growth.

Bottom line: get rid of toxins, and your body can do a better job of building muscle and losing fat. This cleanse—with its emphasis on real, unpolluted food—is perfect for men who desire a more muscular physique.

HAVE BETTER SEX

I figured that would get your attention.

Nutrition plays a major role in virility. It enhances circulation so that all organs, including your, ahem, manhood, get a good blood supply. Plus, it builds your energy and stamina. Erectile dysfunction (ED) in particular is often related to circulation problems; thus, any diet that benefits heart and blood vessels is especially important. Plant foods provide antioxidants that prevent the oxidation of fats that block or clog blood vessels, including those that feed the penis.

I don't mean to pry, but has your sex drive stalled in neutral or slid into reverse? There could be a number of reasons you've lost that spark. It could be a drop in male hormones due to age or another factor; that's something to ask your physician. But a low libido is not necessarily due to a hormonal issue. Maybe it's those few extra pounds—I'm not even talking excessive amounts. Even minor weight gain leads to neurological, circulatory, reproductive, and psychological problems. Depression, acid reflux, sleep apnea, headaches, low sex drive, and asthma are just a few things you'll be dealing with. Reach the level of being clinically obese, and your chances of infertility, erectile dysfunction, stroke, heart attack, kidney cancer, and gallstones all increase dramatically.

There might be psychological issues in play, too. Maybe you're just *tired*—overweight, feeling old, and pissed off about it. But why take Viagra when you've got vegetables, fruits, herbs, and spices? Plant foods are full of delicious, vibrant substances that can work wonders for your sex life.

As long as there's still passion and lust in your life, the right diet can help heighten your libido. Here's what to eat more of:

- Eggs, a symbol of fertility in ancient times, are high in protein and vitamin A, which are needed to manufacture the body's sex hormones.
- Raspberries contain zinc, which is vital for the production of sperm, and vitamin C, which helps boost your immune system (no one

wants to be sick when trying to get down and dirty). Not only are they tantalizingly juicy, succulent, and red, they also help to treat erectile dysfunction by improving blood flow.

- Beets spike blood levels of the gas nitric oxide, which dilates blood vessels, increases blood flow, and prompts the chain of events that results in a male erection.
- Almonds contain selenium, which helps prevent fertility issues; the mineral zinc, which produces sex hormones in men and enhances libido; and vitamin E, to help heart health. Omega-3 fatty acids help to increase blood flow.
- Cinnamon not only helps to increase circulation but is also a great alternative to sugar—the biggest sex-drive-killer out there.
- Basil has a reputation as a love herb, known to promote sexual desire in men just by its smell. It has anti-inflammatory properties, too, which help reduce swelling where you don't want it and make blood flow easier to the body parts you want to excite.
- While garlic may seem like a counterintuitive one, this veggie is actually one of the best for your sex life. It contains a phytochemical called allicin, which improves blood flow to the organs. Extra blood flow means more sensitivity. Double win for health *and* sexual benefits.
- Try supplementing with the superfood powder maca, too—it has been shown to improve sexual desire. Throw some maca in your smoothie and have a sexy day!

OTHER HEALTH BENEFITS

Many of you guys probably eat meat and drink beer and consume protein shakes, all of which are highly acidic. An acidic diet promotes inflammation, and over the long term, it can lead to heart disease, various cancers, bad skin, poor digestion, bloating, and stunted hair growth. Among these, the biggie is heart disease.

Heart disease is the still the chief killer in the United States. The Western diet, which is laced with toxins, saturated fat, and cholesterol from meat, dairy, and fast foods, is largely at fault. Meat happens to be one of the most acidic foods you can eat, and men eat a lot of it. Depending on how it's prepared, it may be loaded with sauces, salt, sugar, and other preservatives. Unless it's raised organically, it may also contain hormones that can upset the ability to burn fat. Replace all those meaty, fatty foods with fruits and vegetables. They're full of detoxifying antioxidants and phytochemicals that protect the heart and its arteries. Additionally, they create an alkaline environment in your body, promoting muscle repair, recuperation, and growth. Plus, plant foods contain no saturated fat or cholesterol.

Don't worry about protein, either; on my plan, you'll get plenty in the form of beans, legumes, quinoa, and eggs. I know this might not sound ideal, but trust me that even though you might miss your meat, by the end you will feel better than you probably ever have before. I'm not trying to convert you to being a vegetarian or vegan; that is a personal choice. You won't eat meat during the detox, but afterward, you can—in moderation. I'll show you how to reintroduce high-quality organic meats back into your meals.

Now on to beer. It is high in sugar (like a lot of alcoholic beverages) and can thus trigger sugar cravings. Give in to those cravings, and you'll end up taking in too many empty calories. Plus, the hops in beer are high in phytoestrogens, according to a 2004 report in *Drug Metabolism and Disposition*. Phytoestrogens are natural compounds that mimic the female hormone estrogen in the body. I mention this only because when men take in estrogen, it can potentially lead to feminizing effects such as "man boobs." I know you don't want those! Beer may also deplete your body of minerals such as calcium, magnesium, potassium, and phosphorus, which are essential to muscle contraction, relaxation, and growth.

Are you drinking a lot of protein shakes to try to build muscle mass? Bad strategy! As I stated earlier, the problem with most of these supplements is that they're highly processed and include dairy products, sugar, and/or fake sugar. High levels of toxins contribute to weight gain, colds, allergies, blemishes, headaches, and poor immune defenses. Dairy foods are mucus-forming, too. They also slow down liver function, cause bloating, and promote snoring.

Still not convinced? Consider your lifestyle. Are you a coffee drinker? When you wake up in the morning do you head straight for that cup of joe, then subsist on the stuff throughout the day? Do you go on a lot of business lunches and dinners that include alcohol? Are you constantly busy with work or travel? Then you *need* this cleanse. Your lifestyle is wreaking havoc on your body and causing hard-core adrenal fatigue. Need confirmation? Try this quiz.

ARE YOU:

- Feeling tired for no reason?
- Not sleeping properly?
- Unable to wake up easily?
- Not feeling fully alert until after 6:00 p.m.?
- Getting sick often?
- Feeling depressed?
- Craving substances, such as drugs, coffee, alcohol, salt, or sugar?

If your answer to any one of these questions is yes, then this is the time to make a change. Trust me, this detox can literally help save your body and your health.

 ## Note from Nikki: Easy Guidelines for Guys

Follow these basic tips and you'll maintain your muscle mass, lose body fat, and detoxify your body:

- Eat a clean, plant-based diet. It will help you lose weight, improve your health, increase circulation, and boost your sex drive.
- Drink plenty of water (13 cups, or 3 liters, a day).
- While on the cleanse, remember: no sugar, caffeine, or alcohol. As much as possible, try to avoid social outings for the five days.
- Reduce your salt intake so your body flushes fluids from your system.

YOU WON'T BE HUNGRY

I believe that a lot of men are afraid to do a detox for fear of walking around hungry all day—especially after seeing the females in their lives feeling grumpy from eating too little on a whole host of fad diets. Is that what you're thinking?

Don't worry. You won't feel hungry. This is not a fast or a liquid diet—both of which can feel like a shock treatment, leaving you zapped of energy and flattened by fatigue. You'll be eating five times a day. The plant proteins here will fill you up so much that you may not even be able to eat everything listed. And you'll be selecting foods that support your body's natural detoxification systems and avoiding foods that expose you to harmful substances.

This won't be unpleasant, I promise—far from it!

YOU GET TO EAT MORE

I don't expect you to eat the same portions as women; they're too small for you. You get to increase your portion sizes of lentils, quinoa, and black beans by 50 percent, eat more vegetables, and grab an extra handful of almonds at breakfast or with one of your snacks. Important (I know, I'm a broken record): be sure to drink the recommended amount of water daily.

If you're having a hard time cutting too many things out at once, then just do the breakfast for a few days, then add the lunch, and finally the dinner—while you're gradually cutting out caffeine, alcohol, and processed foods at the same time. After you've eased into the detox like this, finally move up to doing the full detox as it's written. The goal here is to help wean you off certain things while increasing your desire for healthier alternatives. If you absolutely know that you can't cut coffee out on the first go, for example, but you can manage all the rest of the principles, well, then do that! I don't want you to quit because it's too hard and never try it again because you don't want to do it or feel like you can't. It's about being better than before—not perfection. I just

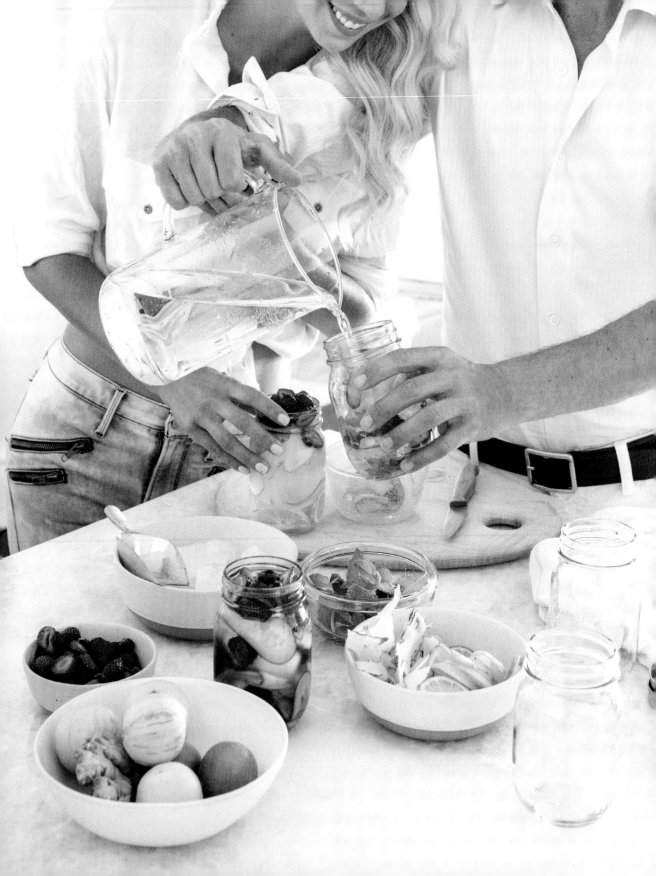

want you to give it a try and continue to adopt some of the principles into your way of life.

In each of the recipes in Chapter 8, I'll show you the increased portion size so you know exactly how much to eat during all five days of the cleanse. I know you'll be pleased with how you look and feel in less than a week.

MY FINAL WORD TO GUYS

Follow my detox, and you'll come to appreciate what the women in your life go through to stay healthy and hot. You'll learn a lot of tricks that really work—and will work even better for you.

Consider doing the cleanse with your partner, too; it may bring you

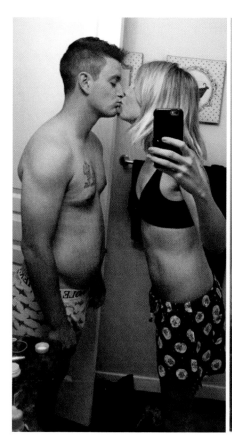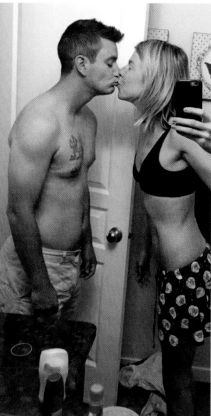

closer together as you share insights and results. Your relationship will strengthen from the support and encouragement you give each other. Guy-toxing can bring you everything from a healthier body to a healthier relationship.

Your body—and the women in your life—will thank you for it.

CHAPTER 8

COOK AND CLEANSE
THE DETOX RECIPES

My husband and I finished your detox, and the results have been amazing. We both have so much more energy and feel lighter! I lost 5 pounds and my husband lost 10 pounds.

—Kirsten

It's time to turn to the cleansing powers of hearty, energy-boosting breakfasts, tasty snacks, and satisfying, palate-pleasing lunches and dinners. These recipes are sure to help you fall in love with your new way of eating. They ditch processed foods, sugar, salt, and additives in favor of clean foods whose vitamins, minerals, antioxidants, and fiber will restore your body to peak health, aid digestion, and boost your immunity. I use herbs and spices in unique combinations, so you won't miss salt or sugar one bit. The recipes are so nourishing and well balanced that you'll never feel hungry, and they will help to kick any cravings you might have.

All the recipes are easy and quick to prepare, so don't worry about spending all your time in the kitchen if you're not a master chef. Also, the prep is even easier and faster if you're equipped with a couple of handy tools. Had you asked me a few years ago what I'd spend extra money on, I would have told you clothes and makeup. Ask me now, and my response will be a vehement *kitchen gadgets*! I'm by no means an appliance junkie; in fact, my favorite cooking tools are my own hands. I don't think you need to invest in anything new unless you're going to use it frequently. A lot of people have cupboards and drawers full of doodads but use only one or two of them regularly.

That said, if you're inspired to start making smoothies, juices, and plant-based meals, I do recommend a few appliances to support this healthy lifestyle change. There are a lot of products on the market today, so it's hard to know what to buy without eating up your pay-check or accumulating unnecessary clutter. I've tried pretty much all of them, and here are the ones I think you ought to consider buying. Head over to my website to see updates on newer versions of products I use, because my favorite companies are constantly coming out with even better gadgets.

BLENDER

At the very least, you'll need one to prepare your breakfast smoothie and make hummus, but you'll use it for so much more. Blenders are incredibly versatile, which makes them ideal for small kitchens. You can also whip up green and fruit smoothies, soups, sauces, and other treats. Blending keeps the fiber of fruit and vegetables intact, which is a plus for regularity and healthy gut flora. You can get cheap models for $20 that work perfectly well; just pick something basic to get some fruits and veggies into your body. On the other hand, I *love* my Vitamix, but realize it's a costly piece of equipment. For me, it's worth every penny, and if you want to take the plunge, you can sign up for a payment plan on the Vitamix website. Another great choice is the Nutri-Bullet, especially if you have limited space. Just remember, a blender will give you different results than a food processor. A blender's main job is to blend or mix soft foods or liquids, while food processors chop, shred, grate, and mix soft and hard foods, so I recommend getting both or a combination version.

FOOD PROCESSOR

A food processor will do all your basic kitchen grunt work—chopping nuts, shredding carrots, pureeing vegetables, and more. It's destined to become one of your favorite gadgets because of its convenience and versatility.

I've tried many different brands, ranging from low-cost to professional grade, and each has its place. Some features you won't necessarily need; others can really make life easier, depending on what you're making or the quantity. There are mini-models that blend sauces and chop nuts in smaller quantities, and larger sizes that do everything from slicing veggies to kneading dough to whipping up cream-style sauces. The larger ones will allow you to create just about everything from scratch.

They cost from $100 to over $1,000. You do pay for quality. For higher power, you'll typically pay more, too. The lower-priced ones won't have as many features, but if you're short on cash, it's not necessary to splurge. If this is your first food processor, go for a lower-priced one so you can learn how to operate it and figure out how much you'll actually use it. You can't really go wrong. My favorite brand is Cuisinart. KitchenAid and Kenwood are other great options with a range of features at different cost points. On the higher end, Magimix is an awesome European brand—it's an investment, but one I recommend.

Ask yourself what size you'll need. If you're making food for one or two people, a 6-cup food processor is perfect. For a family, you'll need one that's larger.

COMBINATION FOOD PROCESSOR AND BLENDER

Many food processors now come with the power to blend foods into smoothies and soups, as well as perform their processing functions. Some have built-in blending functionality; others are sold with blending attachments. A combination food processor and blender is among the best purchases you can make, since it does double duty. The only down-side is that the blender won't be quite as powerful as a blender-only model.

Multifunction appliances are perfect if you're a newcomer to kitchen gadgets. They can create salsa in seconds, make delicious green smoothies, and whip up a batch of frozen banana ice cream. Of all the appliances I suggest, this one will make your cooking life complete, es-pecially if you're on a budget.

The Vitamix and Thermomix are the crème de la crème, but, again, pricey. I have a Vitamix and a Cuisinart Elite Collection 14-cup food pro-cessor. The Nutri-Bullet is a great tool for making flours, blending smoothies, and grinding nuts; I haven't had as much luck making bliss balls, banana ice cream, and cauliflower rice with it, but it is an awe-some and inexpensive machine that can process and blend most foods. Other great options are Ninja, Oster, and Hamilton.

JUICER

When you progress from the 5-Day Clean-Food Detox to the Sharp Lifetime Diet, consider purchasing a juicer, if it's in your budget. Juicers don't need to be expensive; however, the slightly pricier brands will extract more from your fruit and vegetables, drastically improving the nutritional quality of your juices. Just remember that when you juice, green is the way to go. (Making juices that are predominantly fruit will spike your blood sugar and can lead to weight gain.) Keep in mind that a juice should be considered a supplement rather than a meal replace-ment.

There are two types of juicers: centrifugal and masticating. Centrifu-gal juicers pulverize fruits and vegetables into pulp with a cutting blade. They then spin the food at a high speed in order to separate the juice from the pulp. Masticating juicers crush the produce with an attach-ment that squeezes the juice out through a screen, while the pulp is funneled through a separate opening. Masticating juicers tend to main-tain vital plant enzymes that can be destroyed by a centrifugal juicer's high-speed processing. Also, masticating juicers handle leafy greens, wheatgrass, and living sprouts exceptionally well, whereas centrifugal juicers cannot easily process their fiber but are perfect for cucumbers, celery, fruit, and produce with a high water content.

The manual Lexen Healthy Juicer is a great masticating brand, while the Prima PJE020 Juice Extractor is a fabulous centrifugal juicer, and both cost under $100. I personally like the Omega VRT350HD. Remember, the more you use your kitchen equipment, the better an investment it is.

Juicers in general take up more space in your kitchen, not to mention they can be a pain in the butt to clean, but they are worth it if you love juicing or live somewhere where fresh juice is tough to find.

CUTLERY AND DISHES

Good knives are key. You don't need to spend tons of money here, but you should invest in a paring knife, a chef's knife, and a carving knife, which will make your life *so* much easier. Don't worry so much about getting a super-expensive brand (the $30 ones are totally fine), but don't get the cheapest ones, either. My favorites are Maxwell & Williams and KitchenAid.

And hear me out: your dishware makes a difference. It can enhance your meals and make them more appealing. I recommend serving your food on white plates to accent the colors. Use smaller plates, too, to control portion size. IKEA and Target sell attractive dishes that are relatively cheap.

SPIRALIZER

The spiralizer is a vegetable lover's dream gadget that turns raw fruits and vegetables like zucchini, carrots, and cucumbers into spaghetti-like ribbons or noodles. I have the Paderno brand, which I bought online for $30 and highly recommend. If you have kids (or a hubby) who don't like

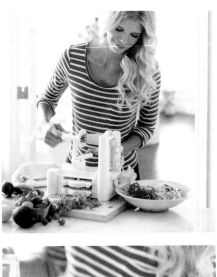

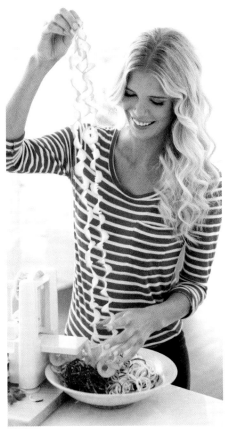

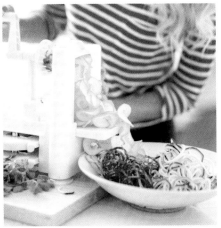

their veggies, start working this puppy and see how much they start to enjoy helping you with meal prep.

POTS AND PANS

This may be a bit controversial, but I do believe in using nonstick cookware. There's nothing worse than having to scrub some stubborn eggs or a stir-fry from a pan. Most nonstick pans use a Teflon coating, and manufacturers have improved the bonding so that it does not flake off like it used to. Nonstick coatings can make your life easier, and you'll use less fat while cooking in them. If you take good care of this cookware, the surfaces will stay intact for years. Use utensils designed specifically for nonstick coatings—never metal!—to help preserve them.

My favorite cookware is copper. It is typically lined with a coating of stainless steel and is the best heat conductor, meaning it heats quickly and evenly, making it great for cooking delicate foods and sauces. Copper cookware is pricier than other choices. However, if you are new to cooking, opt for the nonstick cookware or stainless-steel pots and pans.

Ultimately, do what feels right to you. I want to give you the facts to help you make informed decisions and get your cooking journey off to a positive start, but there's no right or wrong. Once you get comfortable with the appliances and tools you've chosen, you'll be a whiz in the kitchen.

One final note: If you're looking at what you'll need to prepare these recipes or thinking about buying something shiny and new, consider how often you'll use that gadget or cookware. If your answer is "all the time," buy the best you can afford, one that will last and become your lifelong kitchen helper.

Now . . . let's cook—and cleanse.

DETOX SMOOTHIE

(1 SERVING)

Ingredients:

1 cup (packed) fresh spinach
1 cup berries of your choice
¼ cup uncooked oats
12 almonds

½ teaspoon cinnamon
¼ teaspoon turmeric
Small handful fresh mint

Directions:

1. Place all ingredients in a blender.
2. Add 1 cup cold water with ice in it, and blend well.

Tip: If you don't have much time in the mornings, put all the smoothie ingredients, except the water and ice, in a zip-top bag and place in your freezer the night before. The next morning, empty into your blender along with water and ice.

Each day you make the smoothie, try a different type of berry, as this will change the taste and color slightly.

Guy-Tox Serving Size: Use 1½ cups (packed) spinach, 1½ cups berries, and ½ cup uncooked oats.

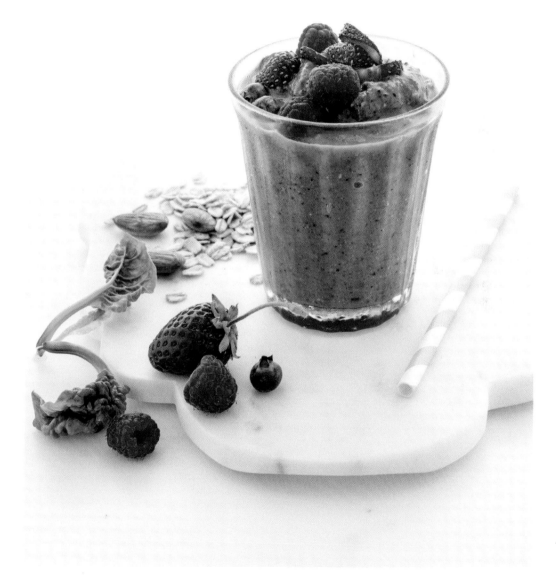

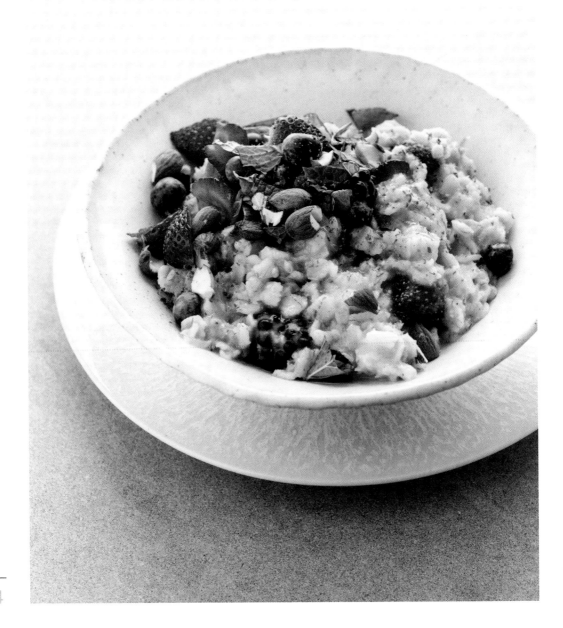

ENERGIZING OATS

(1 SERVING)

Ingredients:

¼ cup uncooked oats

1 cup berries of your choice

12 whole almonds

½ teaspoon cinnamon

Mint leaves (for garnish)

Directions:

1. Add the oats and berries to a bowl with ½ cup water. Microwave on high for 2 minutes. Remove and stir.

2. Top with almonds, cinnamon, and chopped mint.

Tip: You can also cook the oatmeal on medium-low heat on your stove. This option takes a few minutes longer but is the healthier way to cook. You can also cook the oats, then add the berries afterward.

Guy-Tox Serving Size: Use ½ cup uncooked oats and 1½ cups berries. Add more water as necessary.

 Note from Nikki: Cha-Cha-Cha Chia!

I love to put chia seeds in my smoothie, oatmeal, and other breakfast recipes. They're a high-fiber, super-filling source of extra nutrition. They're optional, but if you do use them, all you need is 1 tablespoon per day.

LOVE PANCAKES

(1 SERVING)

Ingredients:

¼ cup uncooked oats
1 whole egg
1 teaspoon cinnamon
¼ teaspoon turmeric

1 cup berries
12 almonds
Small handful chopped mint

Directions:

1. To prepare the batter, mix oats, egg, cinnamon, turmeric, and 2 tablespoons water (add more as necessary) in a blender until smooth. The consistency should be slightly thick, yet pourable.

2. Drop large spoonfuls of the batter into a nonstick pan, or a normal pan coated with 1 tablespoon coconut oil or olive oil.

3. Cook the pancakes on medium-low heat for 3 minutes each side.

4. Microwave the berries in a bowl for 1 minute so that they release their juices, or cook on medium heat in a small pan.

5. Top pancakes with the berries and their juices; almonds, and extra cinnamon if desired, and garnish with chopped mint.

Tip: If you want to keep this vegan, soak 1 tablespoon chia seeds in 3 tablespoons water for 10 minutes to replace the egg. Combine the pancake ingredients as normal.

Guy-Tox Serving Size: Use ½ cup uncooked oats and 1½ cups berries.

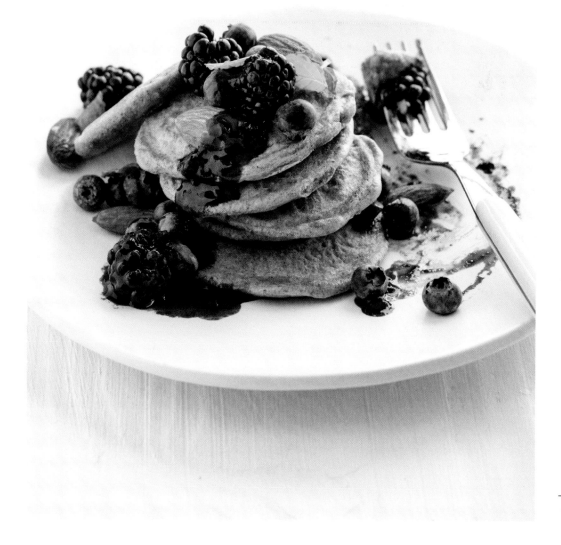

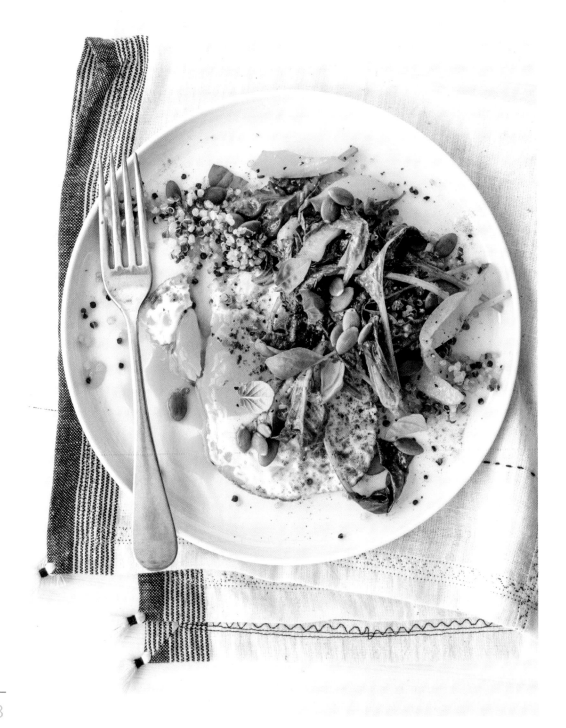

EGGS-CELLENT BREAKFAST

(1 SERVING)

Ingredients:

1 tablespoon coconut oil (preferred) or olive oil

1 egg

¼ teaspoon turmeric

¼ teaspoon black pepper

¼ teaspoon cayenne pepper

1 cup fresh spinach

¼ cup cooked quinoa

Small handful fresh basil

1 tablespoon pumpkin seeds

Directions:

1. In a pan, heat the oil. Cook egg by either scrambling it with turmeric, black pepper, and cayenne pepper; poaching it; or lightly frying it. If you poach or fry your egg, add the spices after you've plated your egg.

2. At the last moment (when egg is almost set), add the spinach. It takes only a minute to become wilted and cooked.

3. Top with cooked quinoa (either left cold or quickly heated in the pan), chopped basil, and pumpkin seeds.

Tip: Add slices of yellow bell pepper for extra color and nutrition.

Guy-Tox Serving Size: Use ½ cup quinoa and 1½ cups fresh spinach.

Note from Nikki: How I Cook My Quinoa

Put the quinoa in a fine-mesh strainer and rinse it thoroughly with cool running water. As you rinse, swish the quinoa around with your hand. Rinse at least 2 minutes, then drain well.

Add 1 cup quinoa to 2 cups water in a pot (this yields 3 cups cooked quinoa). Bring to a boil with the lid off, then reduce heat and simmer with the lid on. Cook for 15 minutes, or until water is absorbed or the quinoa is tender. Remove from heat and let rest for an additional 5 minutes.

For extra flavor, add any of the following: 1 teaspoon cider vinegar, 1 teaspoon balsamic vinegar, a dash of cayenne (if you like spice), or some freshly cracked black pepper. Stir into the quinoa, and let it sit for another 2 minutes off the heat to soak up the liquid.

APPLE WITH SUNFLOWER OR PUMPKIN SEEDS

(1 SERVING)

Ingredients:

1 small handful sunflower or
    pumpkin seeds

1 apple
½ teaspoon cinnamon

BERRIES WITH BRAZIL NUTS

(1 SERVING)

Ingredients:

8 Brazil nuts
1 cup berries of choice

1 teaspoon cinnamon

Directions:

Place the nuts or seeds and the berries into a container, along with the cinnamon.

Tip: If the snacks are not filling enough and you find yourself getting overly hungry, add in a few more Brazil nuts and berries. Otherwise, increase the vegetables in the other meals.

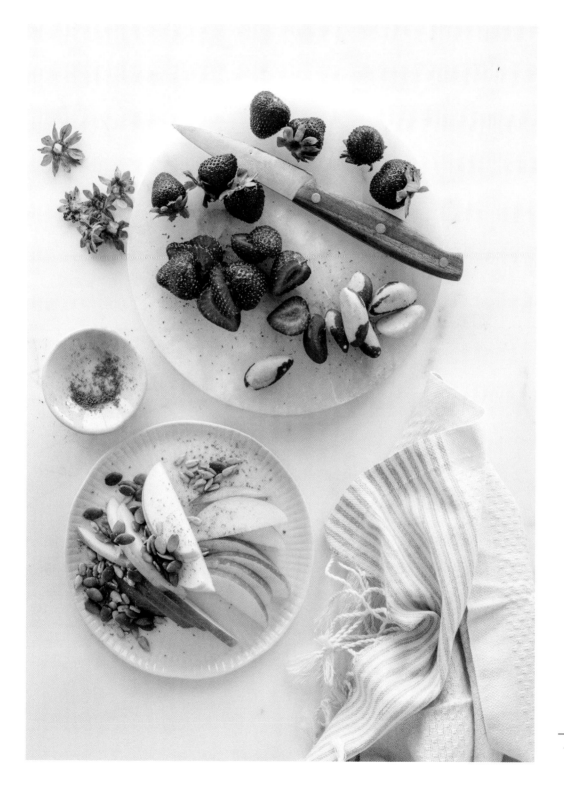

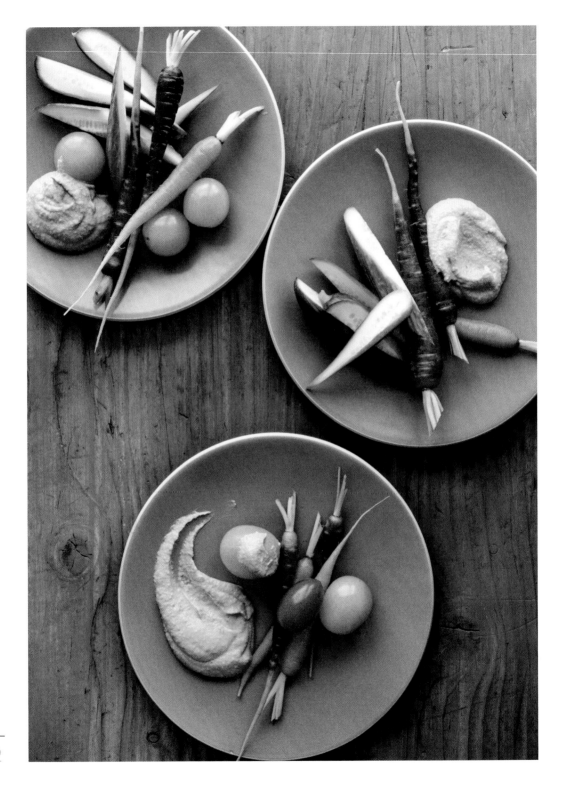

SPINACH & CHICKPEA HUMMUS

(5 SERVINGS)

Ingredients:

1 can chickpeas, drained and rinsed,
    or 1½ cups cooked chickpeas
Large handful fresh spinach
2 tablespoons tahini
Juice of 1 large lemon

2 tablespoons olive oil
1 small garlic clove
1 teaspoon turmeric
½ teaspoon black pepper
½ teaspoon cayenne pepper (optional)

Directions:

1. Place all ingredients in a blender or food processor and blend until completely combined and smooth, adding a little water as needed.

2. Serve with slices of cucumber or tomato or carrots. Approximately 1 cup vegetables goes with one serving of hummus.

Optional: Add basil or cilantro for extra flavor.

Tip: Place the hummus in pre-portioned containers for all five days.

Note from Nikki: Washing Your Produce

Cleaning your fruits and vegetables helps to remove residual pesticides, dirt, and microbes that may be present.

Spinach in particular is highly affected by pesticides and should always be washed prior to eating it raw (such as in smoothies and salads).

Never use dish soap or bleach to clean your produce. Instead, place the produce in a large bowl. Cover with water and add 1 tablespoon apple cider vinegar. Swish it around, and let it sit for 10 minutes. Drain and rinse.

SUPERFOOD SALAD

(1 SERVING)

Ingredients:

1 cup spinach
1 medium carrot, shredded
¼ cup cucumber, sliced
1 medium tomato, chopped, or small
   handful cherry tomatoes

¼ cup raw beets, skin removed,
   shredded
¼ avocado, chopped or sliced
¼ cup cooked black beans
Superfood Salad Dressing
   (recipe follows)

Directions:

1. Place the spinach, carrot, cucumber, tomato, beets, and avocado in a bowl.

2. Place the beans on top and drizzle with the Superfood Salad Dressing.

Guy-Tox Serving Size: Use 1½ cups spinach, ½ cup beans, 1 large carrot, and ½ cup cucumber.

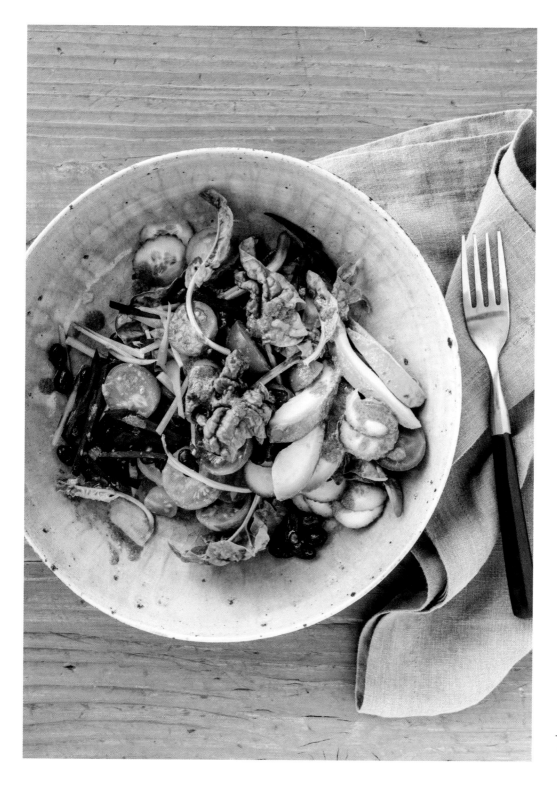

SUPERFOOD SALAD DRESSING

(1 SERVING)

Ingredients:

1 tablespoon apple cider vinegar
1 tablespoon balsamic vinegar
1 tablespoon tahini
1 teaspoon extra-virgin olive oil

½ lime, juiced
¼ teaspoon cayenne
¼ teaspoon turmeric

Directions:

Mix all ingredients by hand or in a blender.

Note: Triple or quadruple this recipe in order to have a large batch on hand. Store in a sealable container in the refrigerator for future use.

Tip: Feel free to add more cayenne pepper and/or black pepper to this or any other dressing.

Note from Nikki: How I Cook My Beans, Lentils, and Chickpeas

For convenience, I normally buy organic canned chickpeas and black beans. With canned beans, make sure you drain and rinse them thoroughly in a colander until all the film has been removed.

You can save money by buying uncooked beans and lentils, as you get a large bag for a fraction of the price. Before cooking beans, you'll need to soak them overnight. The following morning, rinse and drain them in a colander. Lentils do not need to be presoaked; simply rinse and drain.

To cook beans: Add 1 cup soaked beans or chickpeas to 3 cups of water. Bring to a boil, then reduce the heat to a simmer. Cook until tender; this can take anywhere from 1 to 3 hours, depending on the type of bean and their age. Remove any foam on the water's surface as it forms. To cook lentils: Add 1 cup rinsed lentils to 2 cups water. Bring to a boil, then reduce the heat to a simmer and cook 25 to 30 minutes, or until tender.

Tips: Add a tablespoon of any seaweed, such as kombu, to the beans to reduce their flatulent effect.

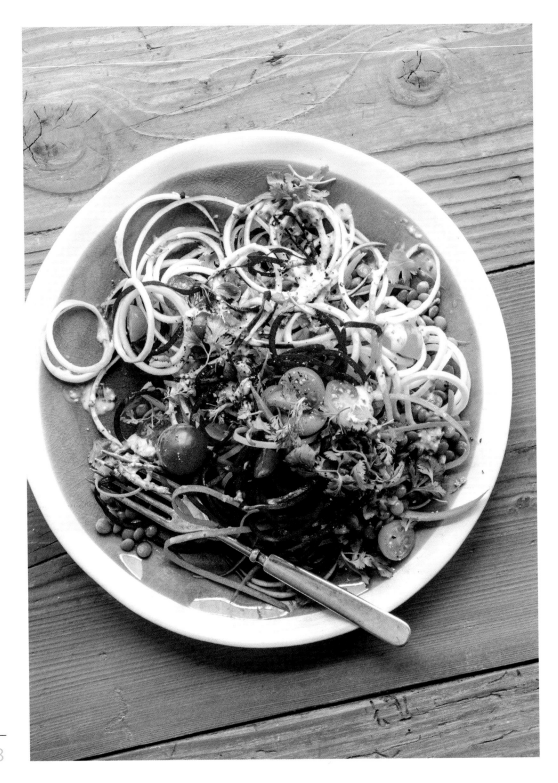

SPIRALIZED NOODLES

(1 SERVING)

Ingredients:

½ zucchini
1 large carrot
1 small beet, peeled
¼ cup cooked lentils

1 tomato, sliced, or small handful
    cherry tomatoes
Noodle Dressing (recipe follows)

Directions:

1. Using a spiralizer, create noodles from the zucchini, carrot, and beet. If you don't have one, use a vegetable peeler to create long, thin strips. Add to a bowl with the lentils and tomatoes. (Note: The beets in this salad will tint the whole dish pink. If you don't like beets or want it to stay green, swap out for additional zucchini or carrot.)

2. Mix the Noodle Dressing with the "noodles." Allow the mixture to chill in your refrigerator for 10 minutes in order to soften the vegetables.

Guy-Tox Serving Size: Use 1 full zucchini, 2 carrots, and ½ cup lentils.

NOODLE DRESSING

(1 SERVING)

Ingredients:

¼ avocado
½ lemon, juiced
1 to 2 tablespoons apple cider vinegar
1 tablespoon tahini

1 small handful fresh cilantro
1 garlic clove
¼ teaspoon cayenne pepper
¼ teaspoon black pepper

Directions:

Blend all ingredients in a food processor or blender. If you do not have either piece of equipment, finely chop the cilantro and garlic and mix by hand.

COLORFUL CRUNCH SALAD

(1 SERVING)

Ingredients:

1 cup fresh spinach
¼ cup chopped yellow pepper
1 tomato, sliced, or small handful
  cherry tomatoes
¼ cup chopped cucumber

3 radishes, thinly sliced
¼ cup cooked quinoa
¼ avocado, sliced or chopped
Superfood Salad Dressing (page 136)

Directions:

1. Mix the vegetables and quinoa in a medium serving bowl.

2. Toss with Superfood Salad Dressing.

Guy-Tox Serving Size: Use 1½ cups spinach, ½ cup quinoa, ½ cup yellow pepper, and ½ cup cucumber.

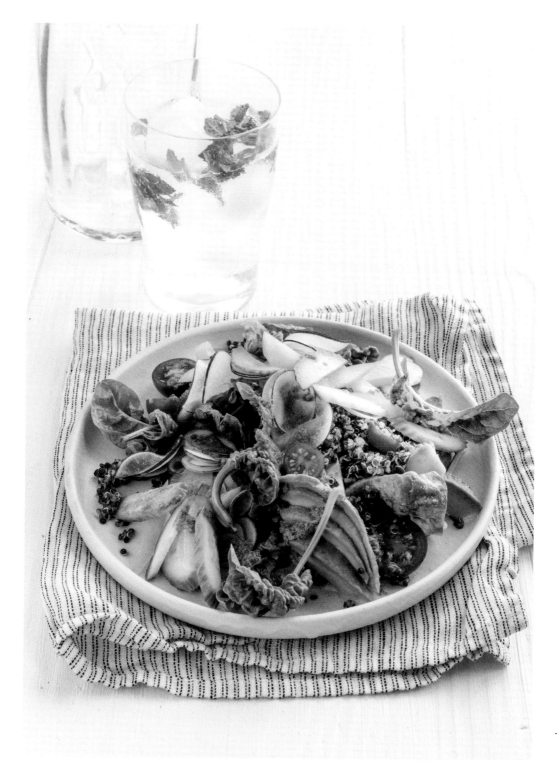

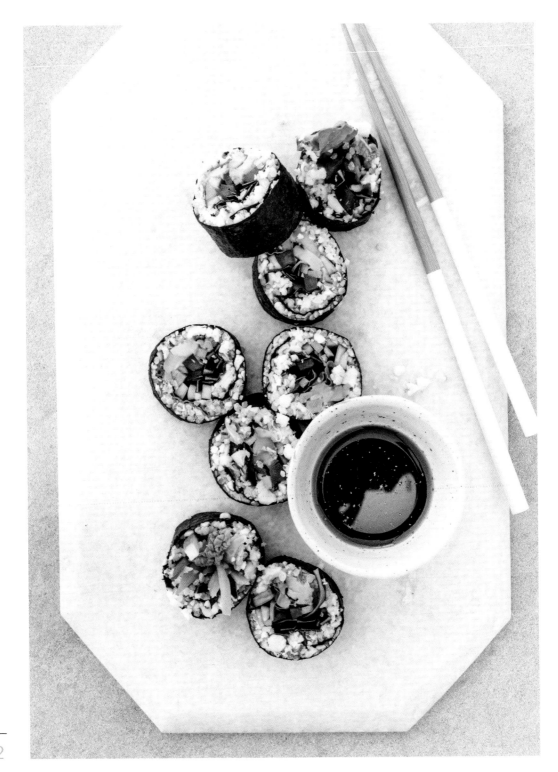

SUSHI ROLLS

(1 SERVING)

Ingredients:

1 or 2 nori seaweed wraps

1 cup Cauliflower Rice (recipe follows), warmed

¼ cup cooked quinoa

¼ cucumber, sliced lengthwise into strips

1 large carrot, sliced lengthwise

¼ avocado, sliced or chopped

4 strips red bell pepper (or use yellow or orange bell pepper)

Small handful spinach

Directions:

1. Place the nori seaweed sheet shiny side down. Using your fingers, spread the Cauliflower Rice and quinoa on the sheet, except for about an inch toward the end farthest from you.

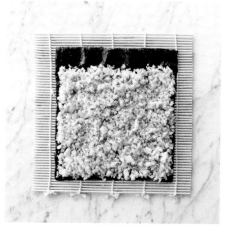
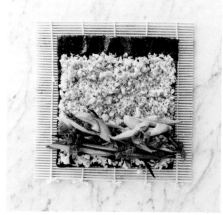
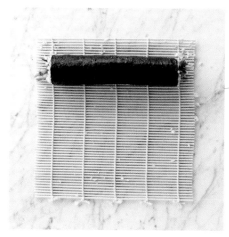
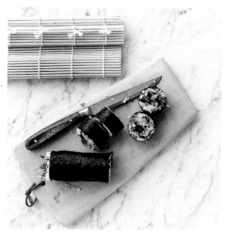

2. Place the rest of the ingredients (cucumber, carrot, avocado, pepper, and spinach) on the edge of the nori sheet closest to you. Roll it tightly, keeping all the ingredients wrapped as you continue to roll. Wet your fingers and touch the edge of the nori sheet that has nothing on it. Once you roll the sushi over, this will seal it. Cut it into 1-inch-thick rolls.

Tips: As an option, add very thin slices of purple cabbage and cilantro leaves for extra color, texture, and nutritional benefits. Mix a dipping sauce by combining 1 tablespoon balsamic vinegar, 1 tablespoon apple cider vinegar, and a pinch of cayenne pepper.

Guy-Tox Serving Size: Use 2 or 3 nori sheets, 2 cups Cauliflower Rice, ½ cup quinoa, ½ cucumber, 2 carrots, 8 strips red bell pepper, ½ avocado, and a large handful of spinach.

CAULIFLOWER RICE

Ingredient:

½ head cauliflower

Directions:

1. Remove the stem and leaves from cauliflower. Cut the cauliflower into pieces small enough to fit into your food processor. Process until "grains" form. Do this in small batches if you have a smaller food processor or are using a blender. If you do not have a food processor, use a grater.
2. Put the cauliflower in a dry pan and cook over medium heat for 5 minutes, stirring constantly, until slightly tender. Alternatively, place in a bowl and microwave for 3 minutes or until soft.
3. Add any leftover cauliflower rice into a container for later use.

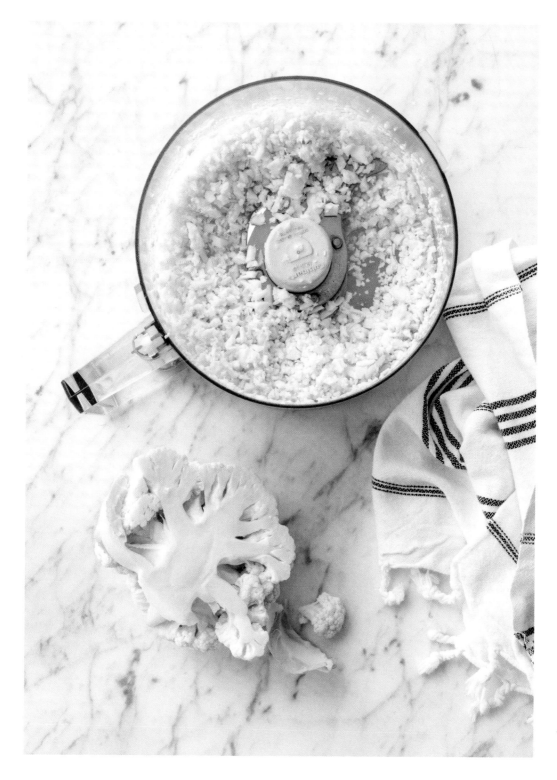

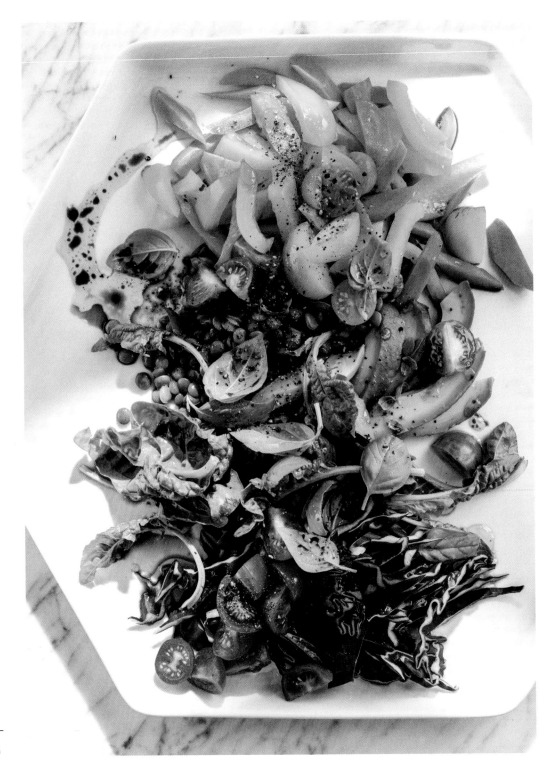

TASTE THE RAINBOW SALAD

(1 SERVING)

Ingredients:

1 cup spinach

1 small carrot, chopped

¼ cup cabbage, chopped

¼ cup yellow bell pepper, chopped

1 tomato, chopped, or small handful
   cherry tomatoes

¼ avocado, sliced or chopped

¼ cup cooked lentils

1 small handful fresh basil, finely
   chopped

1 tablespoon balsamic vinegar

1 tablespoon olive oil

¼ teaspoon black pepper

¼ teaspoon turmeric (optional)

¼ teaspoon cayenne (optional)

Directions:

1. Place the spinach, carrot, cabbage, bell pepper, tomato, avocado, lentils, and basil in a bowl.

2. Drizzle with balsamic vinegar and olive oil, and season with black pepper, turmeric, and cayenne (if using). Toss well.

Guy-Tox Serving Size: Use 1½ cups spinach, 1 large carrot, ½ cup yellow pepper, and ½ cup lentils.

DINNERS

SENSATIONAL STIR-FRY WITH CAULIFLOWER MASH

(1 SERVING)

Ingredients:

¼ cup chopped broccoli

¼ cup sliced yellow bell pepper

¼ cup edamame or ⅕ of a 14-ounce package tofu

1 tablespoon chopped onion

¼ portobello mushroom, chopped

Sensational Stir-Fry Sauce (recipe follows)

¼ cup cooked quinoa

Small handful chopped basil

Directions:

1. Heat a pan over high heat. Add broccoli, bell pepper, edamame or tofu, onion, and mushroom. Stir-fry until vegetables are tender.

2. Once all the liquid has evaporated, add the sauce and quinoa and mix well.

3. Plate the stir-fry and sprinkle with chopped basil. Serve with cauliflower mash (see recipe on p. 150).

Guy-Tox Serving Size: Use ½ cup broccoli, 2 tablespoons onion, ½ portobello mushroom, and ½ cup quinoa.

SENSATIONAL STIR-FRY SAUCE

Ingredients:

1 tablespoon tahini

½ tablespoon balsamic vinegar

1 teaspoon apple cider vinegar

Juice of ½ lime

¼ teaspoon black pepper

¼ teaspoon cayenne pepper

Directions:

Mix all the ingredients together.

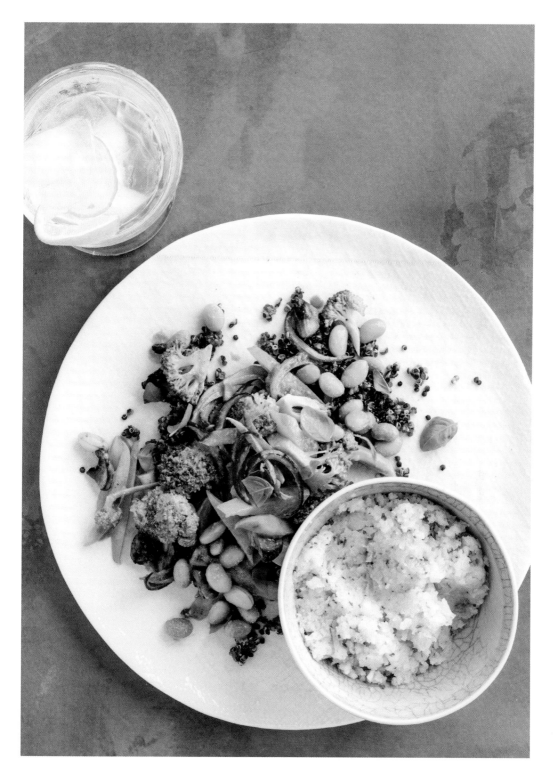

CAULIFLOWER MASH

(1 SERVING IS ½ CUP)

Ingredients:

½ head cauliflower, chopped into
  florets

1 garlic clove
1 small handful basil

Directions:

Steam cauliflower for 6 to 8 minutes or until tender. Drain the cauliflower and transfer to the bowl of a food processor. Add the garlic and basil. Process the mixture to your desired texture. It is optional to add ¼ teaspoon black pepper when served.

Note: Serving size is ½ cup Cauliflower Mash. Place the rest in a container to use later.

Guy-Tox Serving Size: Use 1 cup Cauliflower Mash per serving.

Note from Nikki: Soaking Nuts and Seeds

If you find that you have an intolerance or mild allergic reaction to nuts or seeds, I highly recommend soaking them overnight to reduce symptoms. Soaking helps:

• Remove phytic acid and tannins and neutralize enzyme inhibitors, making the nuts or seeds easier to digest.

• Increase the amount of vitamins present and make the proteins more readily available for digestion.

To soak, add nuts and seeds to a bowl, fill with water, and allow to sit overnight. Drain and rinse.

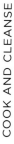

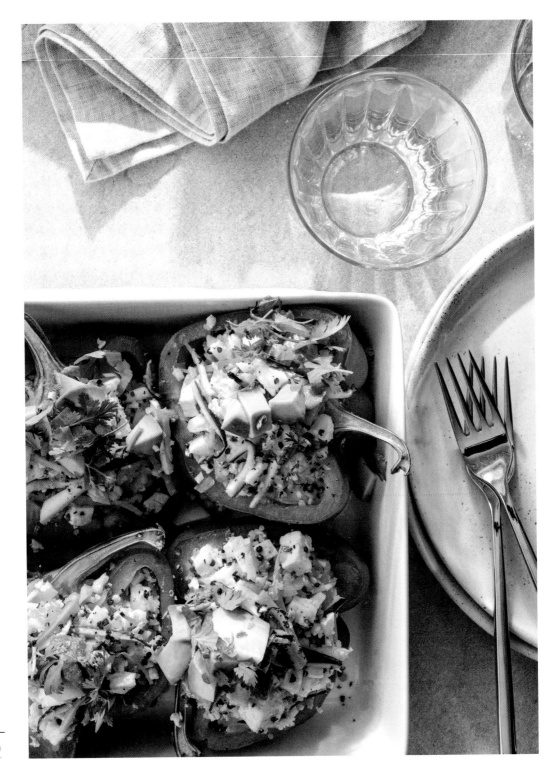

ROASTED RED PEPPER

(1 SERVING)

Ingredients:

1 red pepper
1 medium carrot, shredded
¼ zucchini, shredded
1 tablespoon chopped onion
1 garlic clove, finely chopped
½ cup Cauliflower Rice (page 144), warmed
1 teaspoon apple cider vinegar
¼ teaspoon turmeric

¼ teaspoon cayenne pepper
¼ teaspoon black pepper
¼ cup cooked quinoa, warmed
⅕ of a 14-ounce package tofu, chopped
1 tablespoon olive oil
¼ avocado, chopped
Small handful cilantro, chopped

Directions:

1. Preheat the oven to 400 degrees F.

2. Cut the top of the pepper off, or slice it into halves. Remove the seeds and white part from inside.

3. Cook the carrot, zucchini, onion, and garlic in the microwave on high for 2 minutes, or until tender; alternatively, cook in a pan over medium heat for 2 minutes with ¼ cup water, until vegetables are tender and water has evaporated. Add the Cauliflower Rice. Combine a small dash of apple cider vinegar, pinch of turmeric, cayenne pepper, and black pepper and mix well into the vegetables. Mix in the quinoa and tofu.

4. Stuff the vegetable mixture into the pepper, drizzle with the olive oil, and roast for 8 to 10 minutes on a lined baking sheet. Place any additional mixture on the lined sheet. You want the pepper's skin to slightly bubble and be tender to the touch, but not burned.

5. Remove the stuffed pepper from the oven and let it cool. Top with avocado and cilantro.

Guy-Tox Serving Size: Use 1 cup Cauliflower Rice, ½ cup quinoa, ½ zucchini, and 2 tablespoons onion.

TACO BOWL

Ingredients:

1 portobello mushroom
1 tablespoon olive oil
1 medium carrot, finely chopped
¼ cup finely chopped zucchini
1 tablespoon finely chopped onion
1 clove garlic, finely chopped

¼ cup cooked black beans
Small handful spinach
2 slices of a large tomato, or a few
  cherry tomatoes, chopped
Guacamole (recipe follows)
Black pepper

Directions:

1. Preheat oven to 400 degrees F.

2. Wash the mushroom. Twist off the stem and discard. Pat the mushroom dry, then rub it with the olive oil. Place on a baking tray with gills facing down. Bake for 10 minutes, then flip and bake another 10 minutes.

3. Heat a pan over medium heat. Add the carrot, zucchini, onion, garlic, and ¼ cup water and cook until almost tender. Slightly mash the black beans with a fork, add the black beans to the pan, and cook until the beans are heated through and the vegetables are tender.

4. Remove mushroom from the oven and plate it with the gills facing up. Top with the spinach, the black bean mixture, and the tomatoes. Top with guacamole and season with black pepper.

Guy-Tox Serving Size: Use ½ cup black beans, 1 large carrot, and ½ cup zucchini.

GUACAMOLE

Ingredients:

¼ avocado
Small handful of cilantro
Juice of ½–1 lime

Cayenne pepper, to taste
¼ cup water

Directions:

Blend all the listed ingredients together.

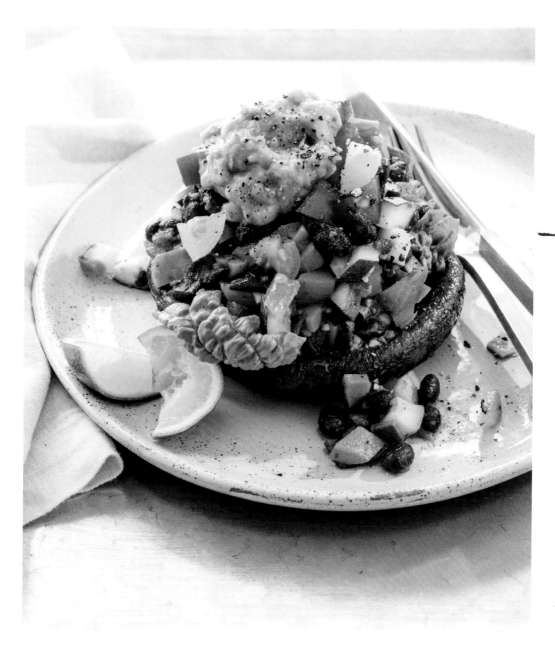

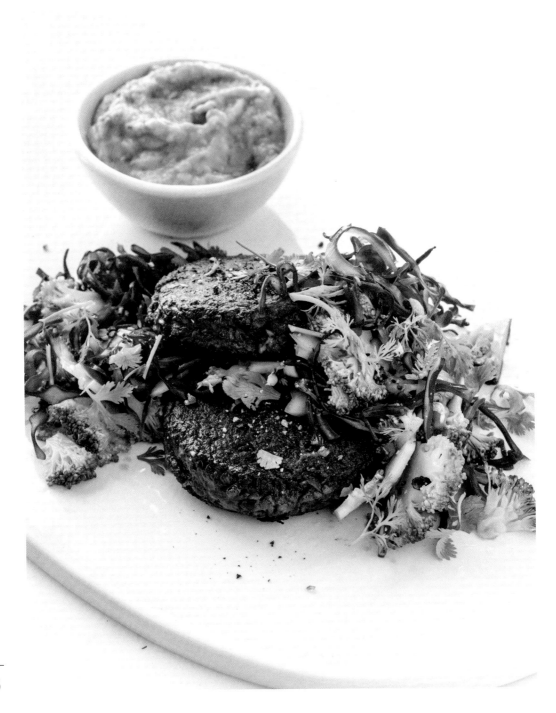

BLACK BEAN BURGERS WITH SLAW

(1 SERVING)

Ingredients:

¼ cup cooked black beans

¼ portobello mushroom, finely chopped

1 egg

1 garlic clove, finely chopped

1 tablespoon finely chopped onion

¼ teaspoon cayenne pepper

1 tablespoon coconut oil or olive oil

½ cup thinly sliced cabbage

¼ cup broccoli

1 tablespoon balsamic vinegar

Guacamole (page 154)

¼ teaspoon black pepper

Cilantro for garnish (optional)

Directions:

1. In a blender or food processor mix the black beans, mushroom, egg, garlic, onion, and cayenne until well combined. (To keep this vegan, replace the egg with 1 tablespoon chia seeds soaked in 3 tablespoons water for 10 minutes. Or omit the egg entirely and cook the chopped mixture without forming it into a patty.)

2. Heat the oil in a pan over medium heat. Divide the mixture into two patties and roll into balls, then press firmly to create a patty. Add to the pan and cook for 6 to 7 minutes on each side, carefully flipping.

3. Remove the cooked burgers from the pan and set aside to keep warm. Add the cabbage and broccoli into the pan along with a small bit of water. Cook for 3 to 5 minutes, or until the vegetables are soft and the water has evaporated. Add the balsamic vinegar and mix well.

4. Place the cabbage and broccoli on a plate and top with the burgers. Top the burgers with the guacamole, season with black pepper, and garnish with cilantro, if using.

Guy-Tox Serving Size: Use 1 cup cabbage, ½ cup broccoli, ½ cup black beans, and 2 tablespoons onion.

CLEANSING CABBAGE BOWL

(1 SERVING)

Ingredients:

¼ portobello mushroom, chopped
¼ cup chopped broccoli
1 garlic clove, minced
1 tablespoon chopped onion
¼ zucchini, chopped

⅕ of a 14-ounce package tofu, chopped into cubes or shredded
¼ cup cooked quinoa
Small handful cilantro and basil, finely chopped (save some for garnish)
1 or 2 purple cabbage leaves
Sensational Stir-Fry Sauce (page 148)

Directions:

1. Heat a pan over medium heat and add the mushroom, broccoli, garlic, onion, and zucchini along with ¼ cup water. Cook for 3 minutes, or until tender.

2. Drain any remaining water and add the tofu, quinoa, and spices. Stir for a few moments to incorporate the flavors. Remove from the heat and place in a bowl.

3. Add 1 inch of water to a pan and bring to a light boil.

4. Cook the cabbage leaves for 2 minutes, or until tender. Drain the leaves and let cool slightly.

5. Spoon the mushroom mixture into the cabbage leaves and top with the Sensational Stir-Fry Sauce and the remaining chopped cilantro and basil.

Tip: If the cabbage leaves rip, just place one cooked leaf on top of the other to create a wrap without any holes.

Guy-Tox Serving Size: Use ½ portobello mushroom, ½ cup broccoli, ½ cup quinoa, 2 or 3 cabbage leaves.

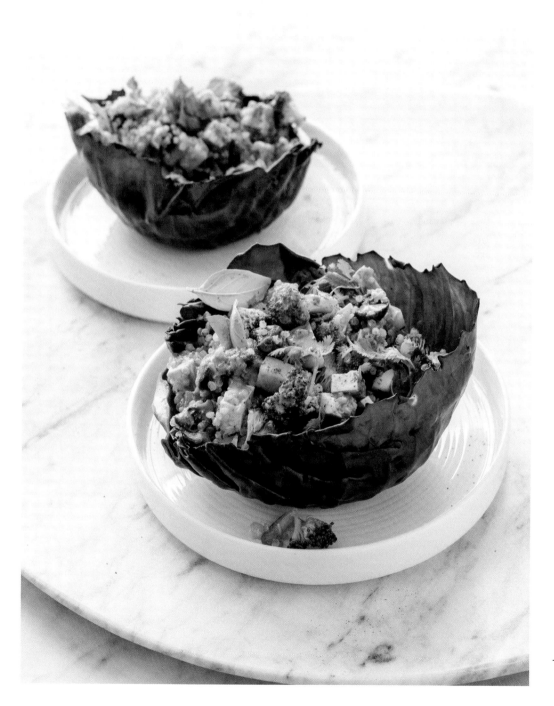

IT'S DAY 6: NOW WHAT?

Congratulations for completing this five-day journey! Take your "after" selfies, weigh yourself, and prepare to be amazed. I know you feel fabulous and look even better.

Maybe after getting this far, you are thinking, "I'd like to continue losing weight," or "I want to continue my health journey."

As you've already discovered, you can shed as much as a pound a day or more, in a short amount of time. You've probably even trimmed

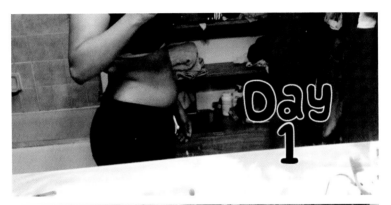

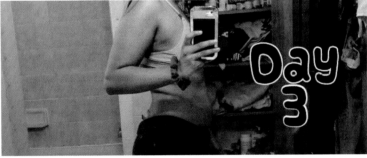

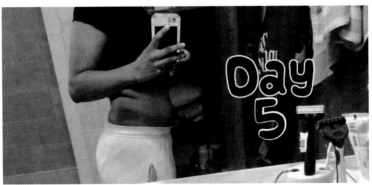

down to a smaller dress or pants size, and your body feels great. Your entire outlook has changed. These are just the jump starts that most people, including you, need to stay the course. Hopefully you will want to incorporate many of the dietary concepts into your everyday life to feel as wonderful as possible all the time.

If you're happy with your results and want to keep going, be sure to read Chapter 10, which covers the Sharp Lifetime Diet. It details everything to set you up for a clean-living lifestyle and will help you achieve your longer-term health goals.

CHAPTER 9

FOOLPROOF THE CLEANSE

SIMPLE SECRETS THAT MAKE IT EASY

I'm a lover of dark chocolate, coffee, and meat. I was expecting to crave those three things, but I actually didn't. What I craved was fruit. I felt reenergized while on this detox and I'm sad it's over. I will definitely be doing it every 1–2 months.

—Lucy

I want you to have the most amazing experience on this cleanse. I've done it so many times—not to mention guiding thousands of people through it—that I have some great tricks to help it work almost effortlessly for you. Remember, it's only five days—short enough so you don't feel like you're missing out too much on life. If you're like me, you'll end those five days feeling absolutely astounded by the changes in your body, mind, and overall energy. On top of that, you'll have learned to love the taste of food in its natural state, without any salt or sugar, and have a newfound self-respect for having completed the five days, which shows dedication and willpower.

So be excited, ready, and on track to nail this thing! I know from personal experience that it can create new lifelong habits that will keep you healthy. They'll give your self-discipline a big boost, make you more aware of your body, and empower you to tackle lifelong nutritional changes.

I suggest that you follow the plan as it's written, or as closely as you can, and don't overthink it. Take to heart these eight secrets; they'll make the 5-Day Real Food Detox easy and foolproof, even enhance it, so that you can stay the course and be successful.

1. JOURNAL IT

The day you begin the cleanse, start a journal. Each day, make notes on the following:

How much water you drank
The type of physical activity, if any, you performed, and for how long
What time you ate each meal and snack
Thoughts, feelings about your health, and emotions (to be completed morning and night)
Energy level first thing in the morning, midday, evening
Any symptoms you experience
What you are grateful for each day (to be completed morning or night)

In Appendix A, you'll find a 5-Day Journal that will guide you through what to record. You can also find it on my website. Not only will journaling keep you on track, but it will provide five days of feedback. You'll be able to see results and progress over the course of the five days, for a powerful dose of motivation. Let's say you want to quit on day three. Read your journal entries for the prior two days. When you see how well you've been doing, you're more likely to keep going.

And don't just take my word for it: a 2012 study conducted by researchers at the University of Illinois at Chicago confirmed that women who kept food journals shed approximately 6 pounds more and kept the weight off better over a twelve-month period than those who did

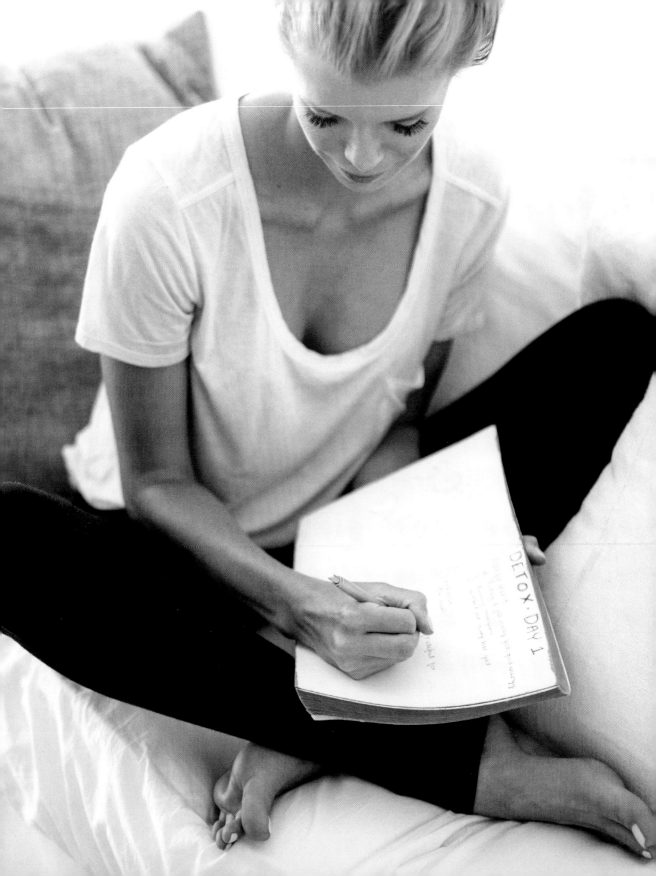

not. A journal can also keep you accountable—and objective. For instance, let's say that you've just finished the detox and didn't experience all the results you hoped for. Your journal will allow you to analyze what happened. For example:

Did you drink enough water?
Did you skip any meals or eat differently than was recommended?
Were you feeling negative the whole time?
Did you go off the plan—by eating sugar or processed foods, or by drinking caffeine or alcohol?

When clients come to me saying they didn't see results, I ask them those questions. Almost always we can pinpoint the obstacles to optimal results.

A gratitude list can also keep you accountable and encourage you to become more thankful for the little things each day. I completely understand that when you don't feel good about your body and your mind is clouded with negative thoughts, it's easy to focus on the bad stuff. Whenever I'm feeling down, I take to my journal to write about all the good I see around me. Often your problems are quite small in comparison to the beautiful things that can happen each day. Reframe your mind that it's not a bad day; rather, it was a *bad moment* in a day. A friend compliments you? Write it down! If you did a good deed, that's a wonderful thing to record. This journal is not just about registering physical results; it's here to get you truly loving yourself.

2. DON'T SKIP MEALS

Many times, we assume that the less food we eat, the more weight we'll lose. Not true! Skipping meals will not only slow down your weight loss but may stop the cleanse from working to its fullest. So let's ban this thinking once and for all!

Science backs me up here. In the same study I cited above, women who skipped meals lost about 8 fewer pounds than those who ate regular meals. And no wonder: skipping meals habitually can slow your metabolism and affect key weight-control hormones, namely, leptin and the thyroid hormones. Secreted by fat cells in the body, leptin controls food intake by suppressing your appetite. Thyroid hormones control metabolism.

Skipping meals is also really bad for your waistline. Breakfast skippers, for example, are thicker around the belly, according to a 2014 study. You might feel like you don't have time for breakfast, but skipping it could be the one thing that's preventing you from losing weight.

Several years ago, the idea of eating multiple meals throughout the day was discounted for weight control. Luckily, researchers have revisited this issue, only to prove that eating throughout the day—meals and

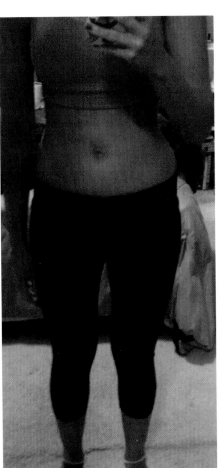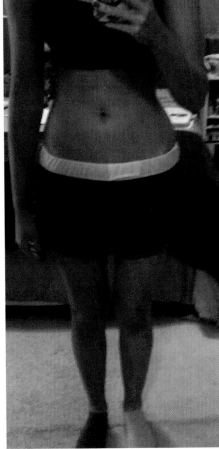

snacks—does indeed go a long way toward keeping us trim and healthy. One recent study reported that people who ate more than four times a day had less body fat and weighed less than those who ate three or fewer meals daily. Other research has found that eating multiple meals helps control blood sugar and blood fats such as triglycerides (which we want to be low in order to protect our heart health), as well as hunger.

Along with breakfast, lunch, and dinner, my snacks help keep your blood sugar levels steady and prevent afternoon cravings. So try to eat all the food required, to promote detoxification and keep your metabolism fired up at a constant, steady pace.

If you've ever skipped a meal thinking that it will help you to drop pounds—and come on, we all have—then it's time to start eating real food multiple times a day to see the kind of weight loss you want.

3. DO THE DETOX EXACTLY AS IT'S WRITTEN

Time and time again, I get asked if people can swap meals and have dinner for lunch, breakfast for dinner, or snacks after dinner. Or if they can skip all the carbs and fat, because they've been told those are bad for our waistline. In short: *no*. My meals and snacks are intentionally organized to optimize your digestion, and proper digestion is key to detoxification. Remember, you'll be eating mostly raw foods earlier in the day and cooked foods for dinner, when they can be most easily digested. Do the detox as written and you'll love your results.

People also ask me about taste preferences and food allergies. There might be a few foods that you just can't stomach. Take tofu, for example. If you find it slimy, try pressing the excess water out of it prior to cooking, or frying small cubes in a nonstick pan with 1 tablespoon coconut oil to give it a little texture before adding it to recipes. Tofu takes on the flavor of anything it is cooked with, so if you've never tried it, give it a whirl. If you still want a substitute, try edamame or tempeh instead. If you're allergic or sensitive to soy, just leave it out and increase the portion of the lentils, beans, or quinoa by ¼ cup for women and ½ cup for men at dinner.

Maybe you don't care for green tea. I still think there's a type out there for you, such as pomegranate green tea, ginger green tea, yerba mate, chocolate yerba mate, or a mix of mint and green (my personal favorite). There's no right or wrong brand, nor flavor. The key is to find one that you like.

Another taste tip for green tea: don't boil it. Green tea should be brewed at 160–180 degrees F, not boiling, to keep it from tasting bitter (a common complaint of people who don't like green tea).

Still not feeling it? Why not try white or black tea? All tea is good for you, because in any form it provides antioxidants and phytochemicals that are linked to a reduced risk of cancer, heart disease, and premature aging. White tea has the lowest levels of caffeine; for green and black, it depends on the brand.

What about decaf? I don't recommend it, because the decaffeinating process removes the beneficial phytochemicals. If you can't handle much caffeine, brew the tea for 30 seconds, throw the liquid away, and brew again. This method removes most of the caffeine but will leave you with all the flavors and health perks.

Maybe you don't drink caffeine at all, and that's perfectly fine. Skip the green tea altogether and opt for only herbal teas.

Other people are allergic to nuts. If you have a peanut allergy, the detox is safe because I don't include peanuts (actually a legume) on the plan. On the other hand, if you're allergic to tree nuts (which include almonds and Brazil nuts), substitute seeds. Suitable seeds include pumpkin, sunflower, chia, and flax.

Many people are sensitive to gluten, a protein found in wheat and related grains such as barley, oats, and rye. My detox is gluten-free—with the exception of the oats, unless you buy certified gluten-free brands. Let me elaborate here, because there's a lot of confusion over whether oats are truly gluten-free. Actually, they are. The problem is that most oats are grown in rotation with gluten-containing crops like wheat, barley, and rye. Oats thus become contaminated with those grains in the field and then again with the harvesting and processing equipment; therefore, regular, conventionally grown oats are not safe to eat on a gluten-free diet. So if you're gluten-intolerant, the only way to be safe is to purchase certified gluten-free oats. These are grown in a field that must lie fallow for four years beforehand, eliminating the possibility of cross-contamination with gluten-containing crops. They're also harvested and processed on equipment designated solely for oats and no other grains. Another option is to swap oats for quinoa flakes at breakfast, an excellent gluten-free choice.

If you hate a certain vegetable, such as tomatoes or beets, no problem here, either. Substitute them for another approved veggie. Just make any modifications from within the shopping list. The goal here is to follow it as closely as you can and make small changes if necessary. Keep in mind, though, that the detox won't be as effective if you begin adding in foods that aren't approved.

4. CREATE A BEAUTIFUL DINING AMBIENCE

The meals you'll be eating on my detox are delicious to taste and lovely to look at, so why not create an equally alluring environment in which to enjoy them? You'll be less likely to cheat or give up if your surroundings remind you of why you're on this path. One of the simplest ways I create ambience in my home is with fresh flowers. Pick them up at the grocery store and put them in a vase, mason jar, or even a water glass—no need to get fancy. They'll brighten up the room *and* your mood. Roses or not, take the time to stop and smell them!

Before I sit down to eat, I often light a few candles, too. This makes a ceremony out of the meal and creates a relaxing environment that helps me clear my mind of stressful thoughts and helps me focus on the yumminess of my food.

Serve your meals and beverages in dishes that inspire you. I have a favorite chalkboard mug on which I can write something motivational each morning. I brew teas in it and drink my lemon water from it. Sometimes I take it with me on a walk. This ritual makes tea drinking an even

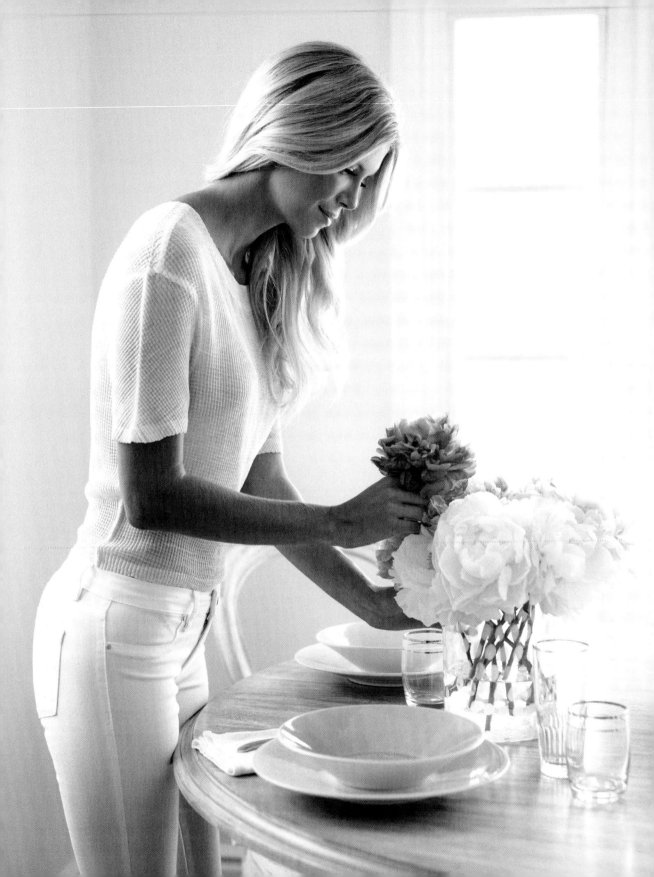

more pleasant experience. Set a pretty table and use nice place settings for evening meals.

Are you on board with the trend of photographing your food? If not, try it! When you know you're going to take a picture of what you're eating, you're more likely to make it look nice on the plate, which means you will actually enjoy it more.

Note from Nikki: Mindful, Meditative Eating

Let's talk more about mindful eating: slowing down and allowing yourself to taste every bite or sip of your food. Mindful eating helps you enjoy your meal, prevents overeating, and can lead to weight loss. It also helps with digestion for more effective detoxification, and you'll have fewer cravings throughout the day.

Every day I see people rushing down the street while eating a sandwich and simultaneously texting on their phone. Do you really think they are enjoying their food or are even aware if they're hungry? Most likely not. Mealtime should be a quiet, relaxing part of your day.

When you sit down to eat, focus on each bite. Savor the taste and the textures, and pay attention to whether you're full or not. Chew slowly, without gulping it down. Chewing increases the sensation of fullness, stimulates digestion, and increases blood flow to your brain for better mental clarity. You'll have a new appreciation for how truly sweet berries and apples taste and how refreshing cucumbers are. Do not overeat. Just eat until you feel satisfied. How do you really know? You've got to listen to your body—your tummy, really. If it's feeling oversaturated with food, or close to it, it's time to put down your fork! There's no rule in life that says you have to clean your plate. Overeating, as well as eating hurriedly, provides feelings of heaviness, dullness, and inertia in the mind.

After each meal, take a few moments to think about how you feel. When you eat clean, you'll be energetic, satisfied, refreshed, and light. This heightened awareness will make it harder to mindlessly go for the unhealthy foods that you once craved. Make every meal a meditation, and your desire for healthy, wholesome foods will grow.

5. CONSIDER SOME LIGHT EXERCISE

I'm as passionate about exercise as I am about nutrition. I highly recommend yoga for everyone, no matter their age, sex, flexibility level, or lifestyle. I started doing yoga many years ago, solely as a way to be fit. However, like many people, the more I practiced, the more I realized there was something bigger there. I wanted to learn about the different approaches, the history, and the beauty in what it provides mentally and spiritually. So in early 2015 I became a certified yoga instructor. I flew all the way to Bali to spend several weeks doing an intensive course with eighteen other people from all over the world. I finally was able to live and breathe yoga—and by the end, I was officially certified to teach it.

Even if you don't delve in *quite* so deeply, there are some specific reasons yoga is the perfect complement to detoxification. Yoga does all the following:

- Enhances the health of your digestive organs, including the liver
- Helps you sweat out toxins
- Assists in weight loss
- Strengthens the muscles and makes the body more flexible, for a more efficient metabolism
- Emphasizes deep breathing to help you exhale toxins and increase energy
- Calms the mind and body, keeping stress and distracting thoughts at bay
- Revitalizes the body's organs and enhances the immune system, for stronger health and more effective detoxification
- Is an excellent way to release emotional baggage, so that you're mentally freed up to do the cleanse successfully

If yoga isn't your thing, do some light workouts such as light weight lifting, jogging, or walking—nothing too strenuous, although a little sweat helps your body detox. And it's perfectly fine to not exercise for

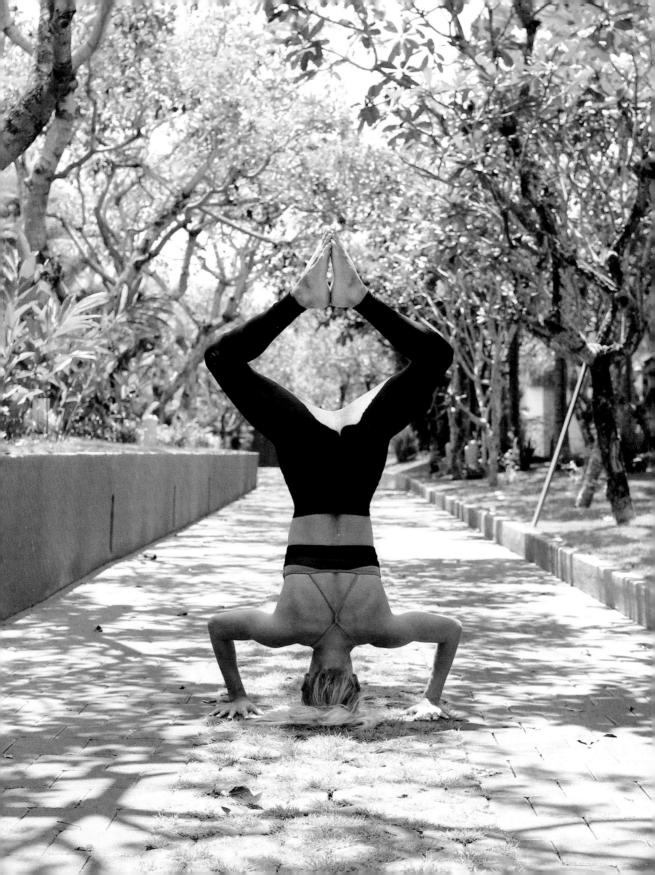

these five days. You'll still get the same results. Your calories and carbo-hydrates will be slightly reduced, and mixed with toxins exiting your body, working out might fatigue you more than usual.

Bottom line: listen to your body. Feeling like you have all the energy in the world and want to hit it hard? Go for it, but remember that an intense workout can boost your body's need for more calories, increasing your chances of overeating or even bingeing during the five days. Your results will be just as good if you don't work out. Trust me on this!

6. START BODY BRUSHING

Okay, now we're getting down to my real secrets. The body sheds waste products through the skin, so it's important to keep your pores free of dead skin cells, dirt, and other nasties, or else these impurities will stay in your body, putting stress on the detoxification organs. You can unclog your pores and get rid of waste by body brushing.

You'll need a natural-bristle body brush, which can be purchased at most bath and body shops, health food stores, or online. Every day, before your bath or shower while your skin is dry, begin by brushing the bottoms of your feet. Work your way up your legs, hips, abdomen, chest, back, and finally your hands and arms. Use firm, long strokes, and brush in the direction of your heart to encourage blood flow and better circulation. Be gentle around your breasts, because the skin there is delicate. It is best not to brush your face, either, unless you use something softer, such as a loofah. Also, wash and clean your brush with soap and water after each use to keep it free from germs.

Once you get the hang of it, you'll see and feel instantly silky smooth skin. Keeping your pores clear and circulation lively will allow your skin to "breathe," improve the flow of blood and lymph, and expedite the elimination of waste products that can lead to cellulite. Body brushing also helps your skin better absorb skincare lotions and treatments. You'll love the results so much that you'll wish you'd started much sooner.

7. CLEANSE WITH A FRIEND

I bet you have a sister, friend, coworker, parent, or partner who also wants to lose some weight. A buddy can be very helpful, but make sure he or she is as motivated as you are. Shop together for the ingredients on the list, compare notes on the recipes, and go to yoga or exercise classes together. Having that mutual support will keep both of you on track. You might be surprised at how many people are eager to try a cleanse that includes this much delicious food, so try to get those around you on board.

On my website, nikkisharp.com, I often do a "virtual" cleanse, in which I invite my followers to follow the plan with me. We share our results and encourage each other along the way. I also offer a private 5-Day Detox Facebook group; participation has enhanced the results of everyone involved. Even after all these years, the love and support help me stay motivated!

8. BEAT THE CHEAT

Even though I've done my detox many times, I still sometimes get the urge to cheat, especially after the first two days. These urges range from chocolate during the first few days to bananas halfway through, coffee, and a glass (or two) of wine. But I also know how to resist. First, I remind myself that I can do anything for five days, and I remember how great I'll feel if I give it my all.

Second, I go for a walk. I work from home and blog about eating, so I'm constantly surrounded by food; getting out recharges my energy and motivation. If you're lucky enough to be surrounded by the beautiful outdoors, go for a walk and see how many different types of birds or flowers you can spot. If you work in an office and temptation arises, go for a quick stroll to take your mind off it. Any type of distraction such as walking, even up and down stairs or through a hallway, will help you avoid cheating. Call or visit a friend in the office, meditate, go to the gym, read a book, take a bubble bath, or write in your journal. Try to get

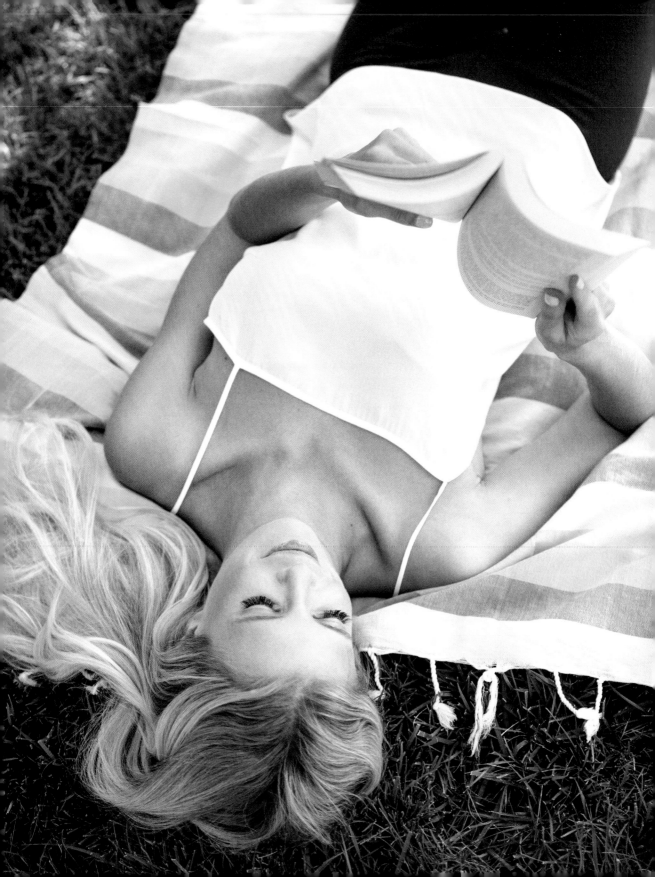

away from the TV or your computer, since you're more likely to mind-lessly eat there.

Another effective technique is deep breathing, especially if you're stressed out and feel like cheating. How you breathe impacts your body and mind. If you feel tense, your breathing is usually shallow. This means you are inhaling less oxygen and exhaling fewer waste products and toxins.

Inhale slowly through your nose, while feeling your abdomen rise. Pause for a second while holding your breath, then exhale slowly through your mouth. Or inhale for a count of four, hold for four, exhale for four, and hold for four; try to visualize walking around a square while you do this. Repeat for five to ten minutes. It can quiet a racing mind and help overcome the desire to fall off the wagon. Just remember: 4, 4, 4, 4.

My third trick: brush your teeth. When your mouth is minty and fresh, you're less likely to eat. I don't recommend chewing gum, though. Aside from containing sugar and artificial sweeteners, it actually increases bloating (because you're swallowing air)—one of the major issues we are fighting on the cleanse.

Fourth, be prepared. A dinner invitation pops up. You have to take a client out to dinner. A relative is in town. Your best friend wants to go out. You have a date. In unavoidable cases, I call the restaurant ahead of time and ask if they have any vegan options. Because you are cutting out meat, chicken, and fish, your best option is vegan, because it doesn't use dairy, meat, or other animal products. Ask for a side of vegetables or a salad with the dressing on the side and no salt added. If a vegan entrée is not available, get a basic steamed salmon or white fish or chicken with a side of steamed vegetables. However, as I've mentioned, it's best to plan to do the detox when you can set aside five days for yourself, without social engagements.

Another option is to cook at home for your friends or relatives, stick-ing to the cleanse as closely as possible. I once prepared a meal for my parents that included my Sensational Stir-Fry; I also cooked organic, free-range chicken for them, and served zucchini and cucumber rolls filled with avocado, julienned carrots, red pepper, and bean sprouts.

They *loved* the meal even though they don't eat "my style" of food, and I was able to stay on the detox while enjoying their company.

Finally, curb your desires naturally. If you really can't control a craving and know you're heading toward a binge, I recommend eating a small bowl of berries with a few chopped nuts, a drizzle of tahini, loads of cinnamon, and maybe some raw cacao powder. I have thrown together this dish when I know that I'm about to go for a chocolate bar or some ice cream, and this healthy dessert satisfies me and keeps me on the right path.

If you find that you absolutely need coffee, stick with black and a dash of soy, almond, or coconut milk. Avoid cappuccinos and lattes, especially if they're prepared with cow's milk. Trust me: I know that the detox can be hard, especially when you have so many things going on. No one is perfect. Sometimes I've ended up drinking a coffee or two, knowing that it'll keep me from going crazy and totally losing my way.

The more often you wait out your urges to cheat, the less intense and less frequent they will become. Remember, too, that while the detox will get you feeling and looking better in five days, it's also meant to teach you positive lifelong nutritional habits.

UH-OH—I VEERED OFF COURSE! WHAT NOW?

If you *do* succumb to temptation, don't beat yourself up or think, "Well, I already cheated, so I might as well give up," and head straight to the office vending machine or your local convenience store. No one is perfect, and for those who have been eating junk for years, it may be harder to give it up because your body is addicted to sugar, caffeine, salt, and other additives, or because it's an *emotional* crutch—it comforts you. Don't skip the next meal. Just continue eating exactly as the plan is written, and the next meal after that, and so on. This helps reset your body without going back into the old pendulum of starvation and bingeing. You'll also teach your mind not to throw in the towel when you do overeat, which will lead to healthier habits over time.

When it comes to cheating, overeating, or not finishing the detox, it's vitally important to forgive yourself. New issues come up every day, and we often deal with them through food. If you go off the deep end, don't starve yourself afterward or criticize yourself. Realize that part of the process is working through your emotions and not putting yourself down. Go to your journal and write about your feelings, what led you to the slip, and how you felt afterward—without focusing on the negative.

Also, don't fall into the trap of overexercising to compensate for overeating. Doing so makes exercise a punishment for eating "bad" food, and exercise shouldn't be approached that way. Instead, think of it as a gift to yourself when you have eaten really well, like after a complete day on the detox. Maybe you'll feel so energized you'll want to work out for the first time ever! It can also be powerfully motivating on a day when you don't feel great about your progress, whether or not you're on the detox.

Be persistent. Not everything works the first time; some of the greatest successes in the world started out as a string of rejections. Stay on course, keep distractions at bay, and if at first you don't succeed, start again. You can do this cleanse as often as you like, so if you don't complete it the first time, you can try it again!

Trust in the process. Remember that radical changes in your body, energy levels, and health are possible, and in a very short time. Every step you take is a step in the right direction, even if you step off the path every so often—as long as you get back on. I know you can do it!

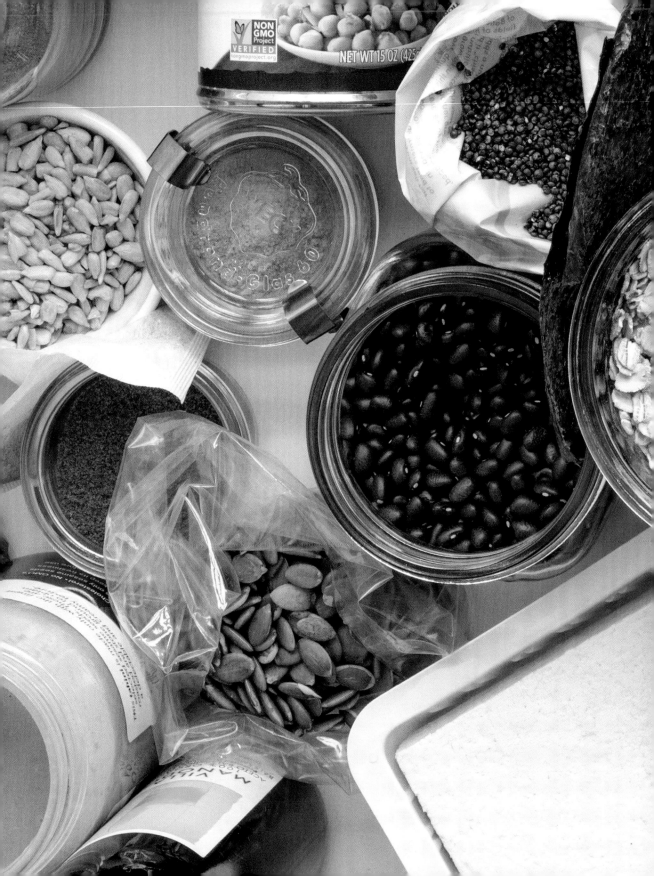

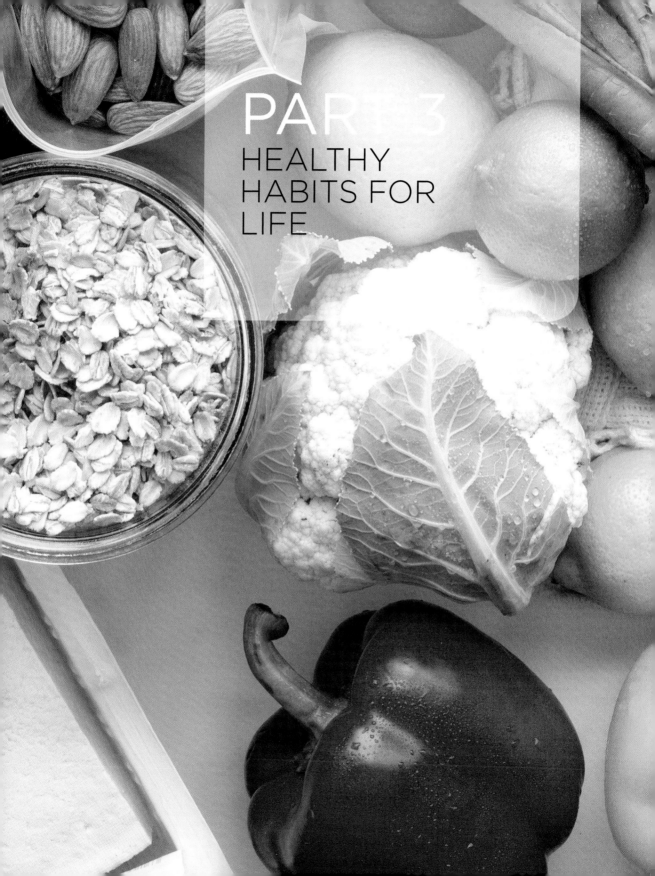

PART 3

HEALTHY HABITS FOR LIFE

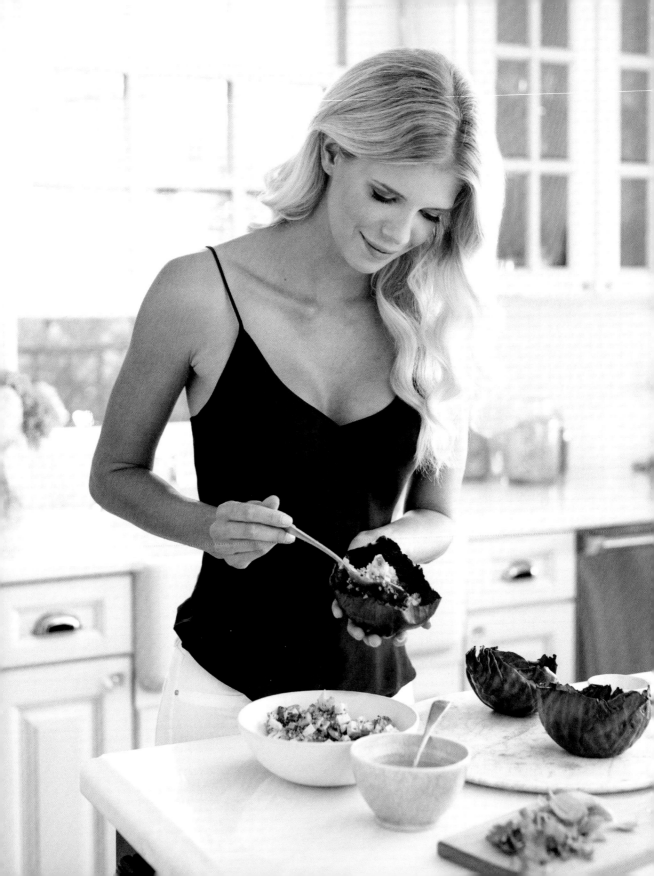

CHAPTER 10

THE
AFTER-TOX
THE SHARP
LIFETIME DIET

I always thought a detox was supposed to be the hardest thing in the world, and that I'd have hunger pangs and eventually fail . . . right? Well, I guess I was wrong. I lost 6 pounds on it by eating all day! The cleanse is an amazing plan that put a smile back on my face.

—Lydia

Now that you've detoxed, how do you feel? Lighter? Energized? Loving the smooth texture and glow of your skin? Feeling "regular"? Don't you just want to keep the party going?

I bet you do!

What you do now is critical. The one move you must *not* make is to immediately return to your old habits. If you're not careful, you'll end up regaining everything you've lost: weight, poor skin, fatigue, digestive issues, and other problems. I know you don't want any of those!

It's time to continue your health journey by following the Sharp Lifetime Diet. This "after-tox" amplifies the clean-eating principles you've learned—principles teaching that what you eat affects how you feel and how you look more than anything else. When you have finished the detox and found continued success with the Sharp Lifetime Diet, you'll be able to further this newfound healthy lifestyle with more amazing recipes on my website, www.nikkisharp.com, and Instagram account, NikkiSharp.

 Note from Nikki: 10 Reasons to Eat Clean

1. Get a lean body with less body fat.

2. Increase muscle, which gives you that tight and toned look.

3. Boost your energy.

4. Have laser-focused thinking and mental clarity.

5. Improve digestion and overall health and immunity.

6. Guard against heart disease, dementia, stroke, diabetes, and cancer.

7. Avoid pesticides, artificial food additives, preservatives, and added sodium and sugar.

8. Protect the environment, since eating clean means "eating green." Because clean foods aren't processed, they use less energy and generate less waste than highly processed foods.

9. Save money. It's actually easier on your bank account to eat clean. Pre-packaged food or fast food can come with a hefty price tag. For the cost of takeout, you could prepare a large pot of soup that yields at least a half-dozen healthy, satisfying meals.

10. Sustain a healthy lifestyle. Unlike fad diets, clean eating is for life. You don't "go on" a clean-eating diet—you eat clean all the time.

MAKING THE TRANSITION

Progressing from the cleanse to the after-tox is a little like driving through a school zone at a careful 20 mph, then accelerating to the normal speed limit. You don't just gun it and zoom up to 40 or 45 mph. You might hit the car in front of you! No, you slowly and steadily accelerate. Now it's time to *gradually* ease into a longer-term clean diet.

During my detox, your body became accustomed to clean, nutritious foods. If you try to reintroduce lots of stuff all at once, you may find it

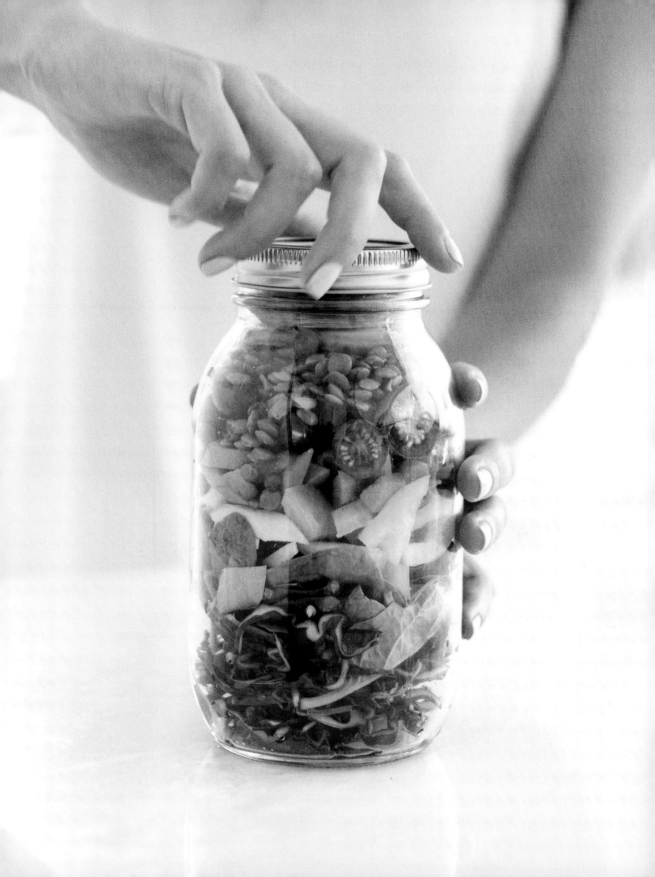

difficult to digest. So for two to three days, I suggest that you build a bridge to the Sharp Lifetime Diet by adding one or two new clean foods each day and continuing to follow certain cleanse protocols. For example:

- Begin each day with warm lemonade. Keep drinking your cup of hot water and lemon juice every morning. It's refreshing and cleansing for your liver. Plus, it energizes your system and helps to reduce toxins on a daily basis.
- Enjoy your favorite detox breakfasts, such as the Breakfast Smoothie or the Energizing Oats, both of which are ideal for every day.
- For lunch, have a raw salad, but add organic chicken or salmon— about 4 ounces, a piece the size of your palm.
- Snack on fruit twice a day. For the transition, I suggest sticking to mostly low-sugar fruits, especially ones with high antioxidant levels, such as blueberries, strawberries, blackberries, and apples.
- Continue to prepare the cleanse dinners, such as the Sensational Stir-Fry, but add some organic beef or chicken.
- For dinner, have a cooked green vegetable (spinach, broccoli, Brussels sprouts, or green beans), a yellow-orange vegetable such as a sweet potato or winter squash, and a protein, such as organic chicken or fish (about 4 ounces) or a vegetarian protein such as black beans or quinoa (½ cup to 1 cup).
- Continue to stay hydrated by drinking 2 to 3 liters of water daily. Once you've got into the habit of drinking more water, you'll notice how much better you feel and want to keep going.
- Avoid dairy, gluten-containing foods, refined sugar, caffeine, and alcohol.

After two or three days, you'll be ready to reintroduce even more foods and incorporate a plan that you can use for life.

IF YOU WANT TO CONTINUE THE CLEANSE

You want to stay on the detox longer than five days? That's great—go for it! What I suggest, however, is that you add in additional fruits and veggies to keep things interesting. Here's an example of how to do that with Energizing Oats and the Superfood Salad. Keep the portion sizes the same.

ENERGIZING OATS

(1 SERVING)

Ingredients:

¼ cup uncooked oats
1 cup chopped mango, banana, kiwi, or pear
12 cashews

½ cup water
½ teaspoon cinnamon
Mint leaves (for garnish)

SUPERFOOD SALAD

(1 SERVING)

Ingredients:

1 cup chopped kale or arugula
1 medium carrot, shredded
¼ cup sweet potato, steamed and dried

1 medium tomato, chopped
¼ cup shredded raw beets
¼ avocado, sliced
¼ cup cooked black beans

As you see, it's really easy to make swaps. This strategy will keep you on the plan while adding in more colors, textures, tastes, and nutrients. You can do this as long as you want, but be sure to continue to steer clear of salt, sugar, coffee, alcohol, and other no-nos (if you are continuing the cleanse).

If you keep going, you'll see additional results. Once you're ready to take the next step, start the Sharp Lifetime Diet for a lifetime of clean living.

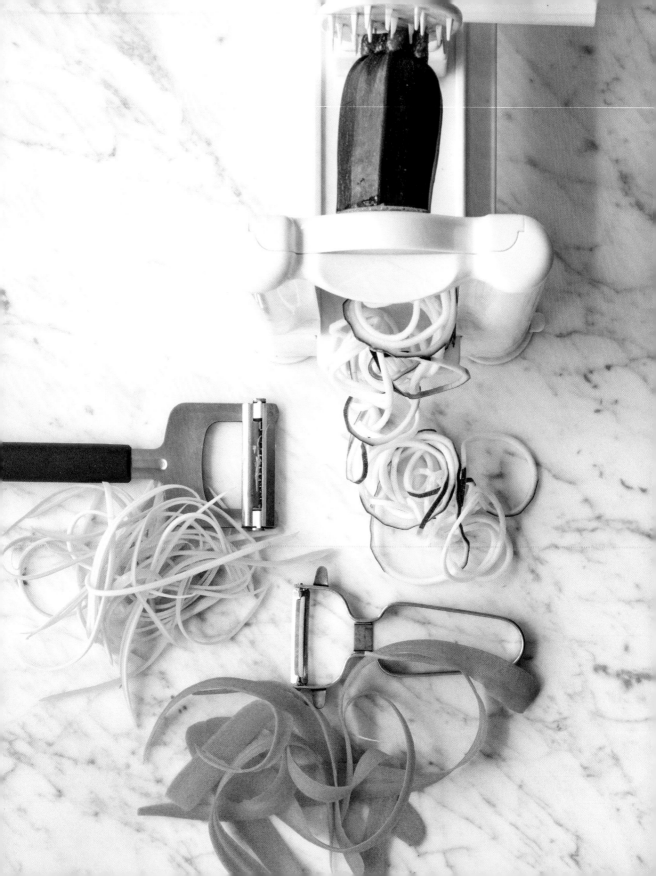

AFTER-TOX: THE SHARP LIFETIME DIET

Begin to focus on expanding your diet and following a long-term, clean-eating plan that will help you maintain a healthy body and mind. The goal is to reach a point where you enjoy eating so healthfully that your body never gets overloaded with toxins. The Sharp Lifetime Diet, or "after-tox," reintroduces many foods into your diet, including additional vegetables and fruits, grains, organic chicken, low-fat beef, fish, small amounts of dairy, and even an occasional glass (or two) of wine.

THE BEST VEGGIES

Vegetables should continue to be front and center. Now you can choose from a broader variety in two categories: cleansing vegetables and energy vegetables.

Cleansing vegetables supply plenty of fiber, are low in calories, and help the body carry out its natural detoxification processes. Energy vegetables are higher in carbs for more fuel, which the body needs in order to gain muscle, lose fat, and stay energized for working out. They're also high in fiber, antioxidants, and phytochemicals. Unlike processed foods, none of these foods provokes bloating or adds pounds.

Cleansing Veggies

Artichokes	Endive	Shallots
Asparagus	Green peppers	Spinach
Beets	Jicama	Sugar snap peas
Bok choy	Kale	Swiss chard
Broccoli	Leeks	Tomatoes
Brussels sprouts	Mushrooms	Watercress
Cabbage	Okra	Zucchini
Cauliflower	Onion	
Celery	Peppers	
Cucumbers	Radicchio	
Eggplant	Radishes	

Serving size for cleansing vegetables: At least 1 cup or more per serving, and 3 servings a day. Feel free to eat liberally from this list! The more you eat, the better you'll feel and the more amazing your results.

Tip: Try to include greens in most meals, even breakfast. Start your day with a green smoothie, like my Killer Kale (recipe on page 246), or have one for a snack.

Energy Veggies

Corn	Pumpkin	Winter squash
Parsnips	Sweet potatoes	
Potatoes	or yams	

Serving size for energy vegetables: 1 to 2 servings a day. A serving consists of 1 medium potato or sweet potato or ½ cup corn, mashed parsnips, pumpkin, and winter squash. Men should double these serving sizes.

Tip: Among energy veggies, my favorite is the sweet potato. It's the perfect choice after a workout because it is high in potassium, which helps soothe sore muscles and maintain the right balance of fluids. My favorite way to have them: mashed! Simply slice and boil the potatoes and then drain. Add black pepper and a pinch of sea salt, then mash the potato until it has no lumps. Don't be tempted to add butter, ghee, or anything else. It's yummy *au naturel*!

THE BEST FRUITS

You can now eat a wider assortment of fruits, including bananas, cherries, oranges, peaches, pears, grapefruits, and tropical fruits, among others. Fruit helps banish cravings for processed sugar and keeps you satisfied.

Years ago, when I was learning to eat clean, I'd have fruit in unlimited amounts to avoid junk food and sugary pastries. I told myself that I could have whatever fruit I wanted, whatever time of day, as long as it was when I was craving something sweet. Within two weeks, all I desired was fresh fruit. I started making hollowed-out watermelon filled with melon balls and tossing some mango or papaya into my smoothies. With these treats, my cravings have *mostly* disappeared (I'm only human, after all).

I recommend that you eat fruit first thing in the morning in a green smoothie. That way, you get in veggies and fruit and supply yourself with natural energy for the day. But have fruit later in the day, too! You may hear that this is bad for you because it increases food combining in the body. I say, skip this thinking. Fruit does a great job banishing cravings and helps with that 3:00 p.m. slump. Instead of grabbing a coffee, go for the fruit bowl (something I hope you learned during the detox). Don't worry about the sugar content; it's all natural sugar that your body needs.

If you typically exercise after work, a banana is a perfect energizing snack because it contains high amounts of easily digestible sugar. I also recommend a small bowl of fruit and cinnamon after dinner to fight off any stubborn cravings. Go for:

Apples	Kiwis	Pears
Apricots	Lemons	Pineapple
Bananas	Limes	Plums
Blackberries	Mangoes	Raspberries
Blueberries	Melon	Strawberries
Cherries	Nectarines	Tangerines
Figs, fresh or dried	Oranges	Watermelon
Grapefruit	Papayas	
Grapes	Peaches	

Serving size: 1 to 3 servings a day. A serving is 1 whole fruit, 1 cup berries, 1 cup pineapple or mango chunks, or 1 large wedge watermelon.

Tips:

• Low-sugar fruits include berries, apples, pears, and peaches. These are the best fruits to eat on a daily basis. Blueberries are good for your heart and help to prevent diabetes.

• Mangoes help break down fatty food, thanks to their natural enzymes. Pineapple is full of enzymes too, such as bromelain, which helps digest proteins; this fruit also helps relieve arthritic pain.

- Fruits such as apples, pears, avocados, berries, oranges, and dried fruits are all high in fiber, which help to keep you full for longer and add bulk to your colon, preventing constipation.
- Grapefruit and bananas are brimming with potassium, which decreases muscle cramps and helps fight bloat.
- Blended frozen bananas are an amazing alternative to ice cream and help keep sugar cravings at bay.

THE BEST PROTEINS

Continue to enjoy vegetarian sources of protein such as chickpeas, beans, lentils, and raw nuts and seeds. But now feel free to add in lean animal products, including organic chicken, grass-fed beef, and wild salmon. You can make simple tweaks like adding chicken to my salad recipes. Clean proteins include:

Beans and lentils—all varieties
Beef—grass-fed, organic
Chicken—organic
Eggs—pasteurized or organic
Salmon—wild-caught
Tempeh
Tofu—100 percent certified organic or non-GMO
Vegan protein powders—soy, hemp, or brown rice

Serving size for protein: Each serving should be about 4 ounces for women and 6 ounces for men. That's about the size of the palm of your hand. The serving size for eggs is 2; for beans, lentils, tofu, and tempeh, ½ cup for women and 1 cup for men. One protein powder serving is 1 scoop; men can double this. If you are including vegan protein powders as part of your diet, I recommend them as a supplement occasionally and not as a replacement for real food.

Tip: Please avoid the following proteins or limit your intake: any animal protein that is non-organic, fish sticks or popcorn shrimp, lamb, lunch meats, pork and bacon, ready-made entrées, sausages, and whey-based protein powders and bars. All of these products contain excessive amounts of sodium and preservatives, which can lead to increased health issues.

Whey protein (isolate and concentrate, in particular) is the by-product of making cheese and a liquid created after the milk has curdled. The liquid is then turned into a powder. Because it's hard to dissolve, manufacturers have to use additives so you can mix it. Ingesting these can create excessive mucus in the body, allergic reactions, acne, and bloating, and fills your body with chemicals, fake sugars, and other unknown additives.

THE BEST GRAINS

Loaded with fiber and antioxidants, whole grains are associated with lots of health benefits, from boosting immunity to reducing your chances of heart disease, certain cancers, and even diabetes.

Cooked grains keep in the fridge for several days and can be reheated quickly for meals. You can put them in soups or stews, toss them with vegetables to create a main-dish salad, and have them for breakfast with a touch of almond milk. You've gotten to know quinoa and oats. Expand your whole-grain repertoire with these other protein-packed choices:

Barley   Kamut
Buckwheat   Soba noodles

Serving size for grains: ½ cup (cooked) for women, 1 cup (cooked) for men.

Tips:

- Although it contains gluten, barley contains an impressive 16 grams of soluble fiber per 100-gram serving, helping to keep blood cholesterol levels healthy. This hearty grain controls blood sugar, lowers LDL, is low in sugar content, and simply tastes delicious. It has a nutty and rich texture, which is perfect in stews, soups, and broths. Whenever I have leftover chicken, I make homemade stock by boiling it with water and straining it out. You can also buy organic and gluten-free stock cubes from a health food store. Cook the barley in the broth; add in your chosen veggies. I like mine with root vegetables such as parsnips and carrots, but anything goes. Be creative; add spices or throw in some organic chicken. This soup is perfect on a winter's afternoon.

- Buckwheat is an excellent meat substitute because it contains eight essential amino acids, making it very high in protein. Buckwheat is non-allergenic, may help control diabetes, and is great for digestion and detoxification, with an extraordinary 18 grams of fiber per cup. This highly versatile grain does not have a strong flavor and therefore can be used in both sweet and savory dishes.

  I buy buckwheat soba noodles from the health food store and cook them with broccoli, onion, bok choy, sesame seeds, a little chile, and some tempeh, mixed with coconut aminos, which is an alternative to soy sauce.

- Once considered the food of the pharaohs, kamut is a cousin of durum wheat and a nice alternative to brown rice. It has up to 40 percent more protein than wheat, with a whopping 11 grams per cup, as well as 7 grams of fiber per cup. Kamut also has higher levels of heart-healthy fatty acids than most grains. My favorite way to eat kamut is over a fresh spinach salad drizzled with a tangy dressing.

 Note from Nikki: Flour Power!

All flours are processed and can spike your blood sugar. If you choose to use flour in cooking, do so in moderation—such as a light dusting on baked chicken or fish.

The following flours are high in protein, fiber, vitamins, and minerals and are your best bets:

- Almond flour
- Brown rice flour
- Chickpea flour
- Coconut flour
- Oat flour
- Quinoa flour

Avoid:

- All-purpose white flour
- White bread flour
- Cake flour
- Enriched or bleached flours
- Whole-wheat flour

Wheat, rye, and barley all contain gluten. However, rye and barley flours are less processed and less likely to cause digestive irritation; enjoy them in moderation.

THE BEST DAIRY AND NON-DAIRY FOODS

You may or may not be able to tolerate dairy. How can you tell? Listen to your body for signs of bloating or indigestion, and check out your skin—do you break out a lot? After I booted dairy from my life, my health issues went with it. Afterward, I realized why I'd had frequent sinus congestion, heartburn, and skin flare-ups. Only by avoiding dairy could I control these nagging problems (although every now and then I treat myself to cheese).

For those of you who are truly dairy-sensitive or just want to avoid it, there are many healthy alternatives to cow's milk that can make great bases for smoothies or as milk substitutes in baking and cooking. For example:

Almond milk	Rice milk	Greek yogurt (con-
Coconut milk	Soy milk	tains dairy, but
Goat's milk		many people can
Hemp milk		tolerate it)

Serving size for dairy and non-dairy: Optional, but up to 1–2 cups daily.

I love all of these choices for a number of reasons:

- Almond milk contains nutrients that promote ongoing detoxification, including magnesium. It is also low in sodium, sugar, and calories.
- Coconut milk is a little higher in fat than other milk substitutes, but that fat is mostly in the form of medium-chain triglycerides (MCTs). MCTs are rapidly burned for energy in the liver and less likely to be stored as body fat. Coconut milk also contains lauric acid, which is an antiviral and antibacterial compound that fights off germs, and it is thought to help protect the body from infections and viruses.
- Goat's milk is more digestible and higher in calcium than cow's milk. What I love about this choice is that goats are not treated with growth hormone (unlike most dairy cows). Goat's milk is rich in zinc and selenium, two minerals that help the immune system, and it contains compounds that get to the large intestine undigested and enhance the growth in the gut of healthy bacteria that ward off infections.
- Greek yogurt is one dairy product you may be able to tolerate. It is full of beneficial bacteria (probiotics) that assist in digestion and break down lactose (so it's a great choice if you're lactose intolerant). Greek yogurt's wonderfully creamy texture is the result of straining out whey, which reduces the lactose (milk sugar) content. This yields a product that is high in protein, with about half the sugar of other yogurts.
- Hemp milk, made from hemp seeds, is high in omega-3 fats and contains no cholesterol, making it a great choice for preserving heart health. At 400 milligrams of calcium a cup, it is higher in this mineral than cow's milk.
- Rice milk is the most nutritious of all the milk substitutes. It is packed with magnesium, copper, and iron—all important to energy production. It is a little higher in starch than other milk substitutes, and may cause a sugar spike if you overindulge.

• Soy milk may help you control your weight, because it has a lower sugar content than the other products mentioned. Soy milk contains only 7 grams of sugar per cup compared to 12 grams in cow's milk. Make sure the soy milk is a pure product and not processed.

THE BEST FATS AND OILS

I used to be terrified of fat—sound familiar? I was convinced that eating fat would make me fat. Not only is this untrue, but healthy fats have turned out to be one of the best nutrients for keeping your mind and body at peak function. As I learned more about nutrition, I understood how to incorporate it in my daily diet, and the results have been life-changing. Oils and fats from high-quality sources and whole foods nourish your skin, hair, and nails, and provide lubrication for internal functioning and a healthy metabolism. Fat also protects our organs, insulating and holding them in place. Fats are also imperative for brain function, since the brain is composed of 60 percent fat.

Fats consist of both saturated and unsaturated (monounsaturated and polyunsaturated) fatty acids. In saturated fats, the carbon atoms in the chain are fully loaded or "saturated" with all the hydrogen they can hold. Saturated fats form straight links that cluster closely together. The result is a compact, solid fat, like the white marbling fat you see in certain cuts of meat. Unsaturated fats hold less hydrogen, and this creates a more liquidy fat, like olive oil. As a general rule, saturated fats are more damaging to arteries, whereas unsaturated fats are healthier for the body, with a few exceptions (see below). Polyunsaturated fats, or long-chain omega-3s, in particular are extremely beneficial in reducing inflammation in the body, helping to prevent the onset of dementia, Alzheimer's disease, and other diseases.

Eat these good guys in moderation:

Monounsaturated

Avocados

Canola oil

Extra-virgin olive oil

Nuts (almonds, Brazil, hazelnuts, macadamia, pecan, and cashews)

Peanut and other nut oils

Peanut butter (organic or homemade)

Almond butter (organic or homemade)

Cashew butter (organic or homemade)

Polyunsaturated

Fatty fish (salmon, tuna, mackerel, trout, sardines)

Flaxseeds

Pumpkin seeds

Sesame seeds

Sunflower seeds

Tahini (sesame seed butter)

Walnuts

Saturated

Butter (from grass-fed cows)

Coconut oil (extra-virgin)

Flaxseed oil

Hemp oil

Omega-3 oil

Serving size for fats and oils: up to 1 to 2 tablespoons daily.

Tips: Certain fats should be restricted. The polyunsaturated fats listed on the next page are high in omega-6 fatty acids that can trigger blood clot formation and inflammation. They may also cancel out the benefits of eating fish, with its high omega-3 fat content.

Eating too much saturated fat can hike cholesterol in the blood, which increases the chance of developing heart disease. Trans fats are a type of unsaturated fat created in food labs by turning liquid vegetable oil into a solid by bubbling hydrogen gas through it (a process called hydrogenation). They are as heart-damaging as saturated fats, because they boost LDL (bad) cholesterol and reduce protective HDL (good) cholesterol. Trans fats can also trigger blood clots and encourage inflammation, which contributes to heart disease, stroke, and diabetes. Thankfully, the FDA has called for their phasing out from our food supply.

THE WORST FATS AND OILS

Polyunsaturated

Corn oil

Soybean oil

Sunflower oil

Vegetable oil

Saturated

Palm (kernel) oil

Butter, commercial

Cheese

Lard

Chicken with skin on

High-fat cuts of meat (beef, lamb, pork)

Trans Fats

Margarine (even low-fat, low-calorie)

Commercial baked goods: pastries, cookies, doughnuts, muffins,
    cakes, pizza dough

Vegetable shortening

Fried foods (french fries, chips, fried chicken, nuggets, breaded fish)

CONDIMENTS AND SWEETENERS

There are clean condiments and not-so-clean condiments. Some good alternatives to kick up your meal:

Apple cider vinegar

Balsamic vinegar

Bragg's Liquid Aminos

Cholula Hot Sauce

Coconut aminos

Gluten-free, salt-free soy sauce

Guacamole, homemade

Hummus, homemade

Miso

Sriracha

Tamari

Tomato paste

Serving size: Use moderately, while adding flavor to your foods with spices and herbs such as basil, mint, rosemary, thyme, cinnamon, and turmeric.

Please avoid or restrict your use of the following high-sugar, low-sodium, high-fat condiments:

BBQ sauce

Béarnaise

Cheese sauce

Gravy

Hollandaise

Honey mustard

Jam

Ketchup

Mayonnaise

Marmalade

Ranch

Sour cream

Soy sauce (very high in sodium and contains gluten)

Sweet relish

Tartar sauce

There are several sweeteners that are basically clean as long as you don't go overboard. They include:

Agave nectar, organic

Coconut sugar

100 percent maple syrup

Medjool dates

Raw, local honey

Stevia/xylitol

Serving size: Optional, but no more than a tablespoon a day.

Shun hidden sugar. Food manufacturers have become increasingly sneaky by adding extra sugar to products under new names. Always read the label and avoid foods containing the following:

Barley malt

Beet sugar

Brown sugar

Butter-flavored syrup

Cane juice

Cane sugar

Caramel

Corn syrup

Confectioner's sugar

Carob syrup

Dextrose

Diastatic malt

Diatase

Ethylmaltol

Fruit juice
  concentrate

Galactose

Glucose

Glucose solids

Grape sugar

High-fructose
  corn syrup

Lactose

Maltodextrin

Maltose

Malt syrup

Maple syrup

Molasses

Muscovado

Refiner's syrup

Rice syrup

Sorbitol

Sorghum

Sucrose

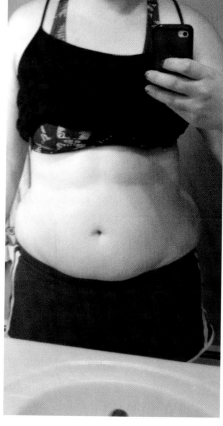
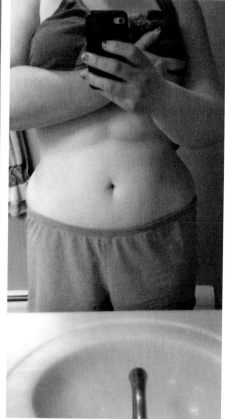

A BIG SECRET FOR ONGOING
DETOXIFICATION: SUPPLEMENTS

A great way to stay detoxified for life is with certain nutritional supplements. Don't get me wrong: supplements do not replace clean eating.

But they'll support your new diet by increasing its nutrient density, which means extra vitamins, minerals, antioxidants, and phytochemicals.

1. High-Quality Omega-3s

Taking omega-3 supplements is like hosing down chronic inflammation with water and thus protecting yourself from inflammatory conditions such as arthritis, heart conditions, and dementia.

The American Heart Association recommends a daily dose of 500 to 1,000 milligrams of DHA and EPA, both from fish oil. This can be safely upped to 6,000 milligrams per day. Omega-3s are vital for our brains, hearts, and immune systems. Try to purchase this supplement from organic or health food shops, as they typically sell higher-quality versions.

2. Spirulina

Of all the superfood powders I've recommended, spirulina tops the list, especially if you're going to use just one. I love spirulina because it can provide most of the protein you need to live on. If you don't like the grassy taste, try the tablet form and follow the manufacturer's recommendation for daily dosage.

3. Calcium

Besides being a major constituent of bones and teeth and a preventer of bone-crippling osteoporosis, calcium is also required for proper muscle contraction, normal blood clotting, and healthy nerve function. If you're like me and don't consume dairy products, you may worry about your calcium intake. (It's something we've been told we are missing if we don't eat dairy.) Fortunately, you'll find lots of calcium in green leafy vegetables, broccoli, almonds, fish, and various non-dairy milks, especially if they're fortified with calcium. I also highly recommend taking a calcium supplement, specifically one that is combined with vitamin D (see #4).

4. Vitamin D

Vitamin D, the sunshine vitamin, helps the body absorb calcium and regulates calcium levels in the blood. Many Americans—especially those who don't live in sunny climates—don't get enough D and may need to supplement. There are five fantastic reasons to increase your intake of this vitamin, as it:

- Improves muscle function
- Decreases your appetite
- Protects lung function
- Helps shed your winter weight
- Can help lower blood pressure

Aim for at least 400 IU a day.

5. Probiotics

Probiotics are the "good" gut-dwelling bacteria that support our digestive health. We all know how it feels to be sluggish or not eliminate often enough after a digestive upset. Sometimes simply eating a certain food can trigger a bad reaction. But diet is not the only factor contributing to healthy or unhealthy digestion. I've suffered from bouts of constipation even when my diet has been cleaner than a whistle. Lack of sleep, stress, and anxiety can all upset gut health, and that is why I recommend taking a probiotic supplement every day. You'll boost your immunity, improve digestion, and control your weight.

Please note: Avoid taking any supplements that exceed 100 percent of daily recommended values, because supplements should be *in addition to* the nutrients you're getting in food, and large doses of some, especially fat-soluble vitamins like A, D, E, and K, can build up in the body. An excess of vitamin A can slow growth and lead to hair loss, while too much vitamin D can cause nausea and irritability. And with the exception of the fat-soluble vitamins, most other excess vitamins are not stored in your body; they are simply excreted, making them a waste of time and money.

Now it's time to get creative. How you combine your breakfasts, lunches, dinners, and snacks is absolutely critical for controlling your weight, staying detoxed, and building peak health. Let's look at some easy meal-planning guidelines that include clean, delicious, and nutritious recipes.

CHAPTER 11

AFTER-TOX MEAL PLANS

The detox was so easy to stick to, and all the food was delicious! It really shows how a clean diet plays a large role in the world of weight loss. I'm going to incorporate these meals into my everyday life and I will hopefully continue seeing awesome results like this.

—Jade

When I was twenty-one, my boyfriend at the time bought me a camera (I wanted a purse). He knew I wouldn't appreciate it—he was right—but he felt like I had an eye for photography. I was skeptical, but I took the camera with me to Australia when I moved there to model. I had one goal only: to capture images of the country, as any tourist or visitor would. I quickly discovered that the photos I was most drawn to were scenes exploding with gorgeous color. Every time I'd look through that viewfinder, I'd see something I hadn't seen before. I got hooked on photography immediately.

As I delved into my health journey and blogging, I began taking photos of the food I ate. Food photography opened my eyes to the power of its vibrant spectrum. We eat with our eyes first, more than any other sense, and a fantastic view adds an appetizing touch that's hard to resist. When someone says, "Wow, that looks so good that I want to eat it!" you know a meal has verified appeal.

It's easy to create that appeal. In order for the meal to look appetizing in real life or in a photo, there must be at least three colors on the plate. Think of a green salad with pops of yellow from a bell pepper, orange from carrots, and red from tomatoes; a brownie topped with a red strawberry and a mint leaf or two; a roasted vegetable wrap spilling out slivers of red pepper, slices of yellow squash, and snips of fresh chives; a fruit salad of pineapple, blueberries, and watermelon. No matter how good a dish might taste, your brain doesn't like looking at beige all day long; it just doesn't appeal the way colorful fresh fruits and vegetables do.

Remember, color is key. And the fresher the ingredients, the livelier the colors and the more vital the nutrients. My rule of thumb is if it comes from the ground and can stain your outfit, you want to be eating it! All of my recipes feature multiple colors. White and beige are deemphasized (except for foods like cauliflower, onions, and potatoes, which are rarely the main attraction), and red, orange, yellow, green, blue, and purple are in. You'll automatically enhance your plate with three or more foods from each of these categories. Remember to count the rainbow on your plate, *not* calories, and I promise you'll see far greater results.

Oh—and M&Ms don't count!

Eating the Rainbow

COLOR	FOODS	BENEFITS
RED	Tomatoes, red pepper (cooked), pink grapefruit, watermelon	Ruby-colored foods get their hues from lycopene, a powerful antioxidant that mops up cell-damaging free radicals and cuts the risk of certain cancers, including breast and cervical cancers.
ORANGE/YELLOW	Peppers, corn, carrots, grapefruit, lemons, chickpeas, bananas, pumpkin, sweet potatoes, winter squash, yams, mangoes, oranges, papaya, peaches, pears, pineapples	Orange and yellow-hued foods are loaded with alpha- and beta-carotene, which the liver converts to vitamin A and retinol, key nutrients needed for eye health, immune defenses, and healthy cell division.

COLOR	FOODS	BENEFITS
GREEN	Artichokes, asparagus, spinach, cucumber, green peppers, avocado, broccoli, Brussels sprouts, celery, chia seeds, edamame, leeks, okra, zucchini, watercress, cilantro, basil, mint, grapes (green), kiwi	The greens include cruciferous vegetables like broccoli, potent suppliers of sulforaphane, indoles, and isothiocyanates, which trigger detoxification enzymes and help prevent cancer. Spinach provides lutein and zeaxanthin, two carotenoids vital to eye health. Greens also assist in weight loss due to their fiber content and ability to cleanse the body of toxins.
BLUE/PURPLE	Blueberries, blackberries, cabbage, beets, eggplant	Phytochemicals called anthocyanins in blue/purple foods are loaded with antioxidants that protect the heart by inhibiting abnormal clotting in the blood. They also are rich sources of bioflavonoids, which fight inflammation.

COLORIZE YOUR PLATE

For each main meal (breakfast, lunch, and dinner), have one clean protein, three colors of fruits or vegetables, and a grain or energy vegetable, in one or two of those meals. I recommend adding quinoa as the grain and lentils or black beans as energy vegetables, because they supply additional protein.

Stick to the principles of the detox and its portion sizes. For example, if you're having a salad for lunch, make it with 1 cup spinach, ¼ cup chopped tomato, 1 large carrot (shredded), ¼ cup cooked quinoa, and another vegetable or two of your choice. Examples:

Breakfast Plate: 2 eggs scrambled with chopped red and green peppers, plus 1 orange and 1 slice gluten-free whole-grain bread
Lunch Plate: Organic chicken on top of fresh raw spinach, black rice, slices of red onion, and shredded carrots
Dinner Plate: Grilled wild-caught salmon with purple cabbage slaw, a medium baked sweet potato, and sliced tomatoes

Snacks: Homemade hummus and carrots, tomatoes, or cucumbers for dipping; my Detox Smoothie; a glass of freshly made juice (use the 3:1 ratio of vegetables to fruits) or 1 piece of fresh fruit with a handful of nuts or seeds.

See how easy meal planning can be when you count colors? To help you even more, here is a ten-day meal plan to show you exactly how this rainbow system works out in real life. The recipes appear in Appendix B, and the cleanse recipes in Chapter 8. You can also plan some of your meals without using specific recipes, according to the blueprint above.

A 10-DAY SAMPLE MEAL PLAN

Day 1

Breakfast: Tomato Bombs (page 235) and 1 cup berries OR eggs scrambled with vegetables such as red onions, red bell pepper, and spinach, with a side dish of 1 cup chopped fresh fruit

Lunch: Spring Forward Salad (page 238) OR a salad made with spinach or kale, chopped tomato, slices of yellow bell pepper, ½ cup black beans, and drizzled with a little olive oil and balsamic

Dinner: Cauliflower Pizza (page 242) OR Taco Bowl (page 154)

Day 2

Breakfast: Superfood Smoothie (page 236) OR Love Pancakes (page 126)

Lunch: Garden Salad (page 239) OR Zucchini Pasta Salad (page 239)

Dinner: Sensational Stir-Fry (page 148) (add some organic chicken or beef strips and serve over quinoa) OR grilled salmon, a tossed green salad, and a baked sweet potato

Day 3

Breakfast: Lean Clean Oatmeal (page 236) OR High-Protein Pancakes (page 237)

Lunch: Superfood Salad (page 134) with organic chicken OR a tuna sandwich made with gluten-free bread, alfalfa sprouts, beets, and sliced tomato

Dinner: Roasted Red Pepper (page 153) OR grilled organic chicken, steamed green beans sprinkled with chopped red bell pepper, and winter squash

Day 4

Breakfast: Detox Smoothie (page 122) OR any homemade smoothie with your combination of fruit, vegetables, vegan protein powder, and a base such as coconut water or a non-dairy milk

Lunch: Hummus Wrap (page 240) OR a portobello sandwich (sliced Portobello mushroom, sliced tomato, broccoli sprouts, and a slice of onion between 2 slices of gluten-free bread)

Dinner: Mediterranean Lasagna (page 243) OR organic beef strips with Cauliflower Mash (page 150) and cooked carrots on the side

Day 5

Breakfast: Very Berry Smoothie (page 237) OR oatmeal topped with an assortment of fresh berries and chopped mint

Lunch: Spiralized Noodles (page 139) with organic chicken, a tossed salad, and roasted beets

Dinner: Cabbage Patch Wraps (page 243) OR a bowl of hearty vegetarian minestrone soup with a tossed salad

Breakfast: any homemade smoothie with your combination of fruit, vegetables, vegan protein powder, and a base such as coconut water or a non-dairy milk

Lunch: Homemade Burgers with Caramelized Onions (page 240) OR a vegetable sandwich consisting of hummus, sliced avocado, slices of carrot, and sprouts between two slices of gluten-free bread

Dinner: Small grilled grass-fed steak, a baked potato, and steamed broccoli with red bell pepper slices

Breakfast: Energizing Oats (page 125) OR an omelet filled with chopped red onions, chopped tomatoes, spinach, and chopped orange bell pepper

Lunch: Asian Spring Rolls (page 241) OR a chopped kale salad with sliced strawberries, shredded carrots, ¼ cup quinoa, and ¼ cup feta cheese crumbles

Dinner: Zucchini Bolognese (page 244) OR roasted vegetables such as Brussels sprouts, zucchini, red bell peppers, and onions with grilled tofu

Breakfast: Eggs-cellent Breakfast (page 129) OR Detox Smoothie

Lunch: Colorful Crunch Salad (page 140) with grilled wild-caught salmon or organic chicken and brown rice

Dinner: Moroccan Dinner Salad (page 245) OR Sensational Stir-Fry (page 148) with grass-fed beef strips

Breakfast: Ginger Smoothie (page 237) OR ½ cup cooked quinoa topped with an assortment of berries

Lunch: Sushi Rolls (page 143) OR a roasted vegetable sandwich made with two slices of gluten-free bread

Dinner: Cleansing Cabbage Bowl (page 158) OR a large bowl of vegetarian chili

Day 10

Breakfast: Love Pancakes (page 126) OR Sharpies SOS Smoothie (page 238)

Lunch: Taste the Rainbow Salad (page 147) with ½–1 cup chickpeas OR a portobello sandwich (sliced portobello mushroom, sliced tomato, broccoli sprouts, and a slice of onion between 2 slices of gluten-free bread)

Dinner: Chana Masala (page 245) OR spaghetti squash tossed with olive oil, lemon, feta cheese, and chopped basil

Suggested Snacks

Each day, enjoy two snacks. These can be fruit, nut, and seed combos, homemade hummus, smoothies, juices, raw veggies, or the following recipes:

Killer Kale Smoothie (page 246)

Piña Colada Smoothie (page 246)

Spinach & Chickpea Hummus (page 133)

Berries with Brazil Nuts (page 130)

Jungle Juice (page 247)

Up Beet (page 247)

Ginger Smoothie (page 237)

Sharpies SOS Smoothie (page 238)

Bliss Balls (page 247)

Desserts

At lunch or dinner, feel free to enjoy one of these desserts:

Raw Carrot Cupcakes (page 248)
Green Tea Ice Cream (page 249)
Triple-Layer Berry Cheesecake (page 249)
Raw Chocolate Mousse Tarts (page 250)

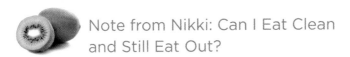 Note from Nikki: Can I Eat Clean and Still Eat Out?

Yes! Going to restaurants shouldn't restrict you; in fact, it should do the opposite because you have all the control over what to eat. Here are my go-to rules:

1. Look for dishes that are steamed, roasted, baked, or grilled; avoid anything fried. This simple swap can save you a huge amount of calories and will keep your body thanking you, since these options won't leave you feeling heavy after a meal.

2. Don't be shy to ask for modifications. If necessary, I'll always see if a dish can be cooked differently. For example, I ask the chef to leave off the cheese, prepare the dish with less salt, or request only half the rice (especially with sushi). If all else fails, I tell the waitstaff that I'm vegan (even if you're not, this still works wonders for getting the healthiest options!). They're usually glad to show me the healthiest plant-based options.

3. Skip all-you-can-eat buffets or establishments that serve huge portions for little money. The food will likely be low quality, laced with pesticides, and designed to make you overeat. Try to skip the drive-throughs and $1 burgers, instead opting for quality over quantity.

4. Order a side of vegetables and ask for it to be served first. I love to ask for some sautéed spinach, steamed broccoli, Brussels sprouts, or seasonal vegetables and have them bring it out as an appetizer, which fills me up prior to my meal, especially if I'm ordering a less healthy option.

5. Just say no to the bread basket. I understand that bread is free, and hey, we all like free things, but remember the true cost: later, it'll cause

bloating or turn up on your hips or tummy. Not to mention that when you indulge in the bread basket, you're less likely to really enjoy the meal you ordered.

6. Plan your indulgences. Don't wait until you order to figure out if you will eat healthy or not. Choose a "cheat" meal once a week and stick to it. Don't order buffalo wings at the last minute just because they look good; remind yourself of your original intentions.

7. Order a bottle of sparkling water with freshly squeezed lemon juice. Not all restaurants have lemon juice (although many will if they serve cocktails), and if that's the case, order fresh lemons or limes and squeeze them yourself. This is a delicious drink that satisfies and cleanses the palate, not to mention that it actually makes you crave healthier meal options. This is my favorite thing to do whenever I'm out, and you'll find me ordering and drinking this before any cocktails or wine, and before eating.

8. Order a mint tea at the end of your meal. Not only will this help with digestion and reduce bloating, but it will help your mind to signal that the meal is done. Ever wonder why mint gum is so popular? Same reason. But skip the gum and switch over to the body-healthy mint tea.

9. Share an appetizer and main course with someone. This will still allow you to indulge in whatever you want, while eating a smaller portion size.

10. Ask yourself, "Is it made with love?" This is my go-to thing when dining out, because if I feel like my burger has been thrown together by someone who doesn't care, then it means the ingredients were probably created in the same manner. Think about when you go to someone's house for dinner and the amount of time and effort (i.e., love) they put into buying the ingredients, making the food, and setting the table. The same effort should go into your food when you dine out. I will never tell you not to hit a fast-food joint ever again, but I will say that when you start noticing how little effort or care your food is made with, you will start to enjoy saving up and spending your money on higher-quality meals.

SEASONAL NUTRITION

I believe in enjoying fruits and vegetables when they're in season; this helps your body sync up with the Earth. When you're harmonized with the Earth's natural cycles, you begin to desire fruits and veggies as they're ripening, and you'll be less likely to crave junk food or sugary stuff.

Eating by season will also satisfy you in other ways. Some foods warm you up, and others cool you down—this is a basic philosophy of Chinese medicine. In the winter and fall, you'll feel more satisfied with your food choices if you eat warmer, heavier, and spicier foods, including good fats from nuts, seeds, oils, and fish. Chicken, turkey, and beef are useful during the colder months because they help energize the body. Just remember to eat free-range and organic to minimize ingesting harmful hormones. They'll also help keep your mucous membranes moist and less susceptible to cold season. Focus on creating soul-warming meals such as soups and stews.

Spring and summer are a good time to focus on cooling foods. When it's hot outside, your body naturally craves lovely fruits and vegetables with a higher water content, such as watermelon and cucumbers. Foods like tofu, melons, and bananas are also cooling and moistening. This is logical and intuitive. If you hold a piece of tofu, it feels cold and damp. Those are its energetic principles, and that's the effect it will have in the body.

Grains fall somewhere between warm and cooling, so you can keep them on your plate all through the year.

As always, the key is balance. Don't go overboard with too much of a certain food or type of food. Instead, incorporate foods gently and mindfully, noticing how any particular food feels in your body during and after eating it. The goal is to eat as seasonally as you can, making sure that your food is organic and not full of chemicals, pesticides, and other nasties.

 ### Note from Nikki: Traveling Clean

I get asked all the time how I stay healthy and lean when I travel. It's not that hard, really. Here are my tips for "traveling clean."

1. Loosen up a bit. You can be as strict at home as you like, but when you're in a new city, part of the experience is eating the local food. Suppose you go to Italy. I know you want to taste the wonderful pizza or pasta (it's a lot better than what we eat in the States). Unless you have a real medical issue, it would be a shame to abstain because you're afraid of gluten and miss out on something absolutely delicious. You can always get back on track when you're home. Just remember to eat in a balanced way, so you don't "throw in the towel" and plan on gaining weight.

2. Select your indulgences and stick with them. Not only do I want to enjoy pizza and pasta in Italy; I also love coffee and croissants in France and Greek yogurt in Greece. Everywhere you go, learn about the local cuisine and what the region or city is best known for. Plan a time or place to enjoy that particular meal. Go to locally owned restaurants, too, rather than touristy joints, for the real deal.

3. Enjoy and appreciate. Never feel guilty about eating something special. Instead, enjoy it mindfully. Relax, say a little prayer of gratitude for this adventure, and savor your delicious meal slowly.

4. Pack your own in-transit food. Especially if you're traveling by air. That way, you won't be tempted by pastries, sandwiches, chips, crackers, chocolates, or dreadful airline meals. My go-to travel snacks are:

• Raw nuts. I love almonds and cashews.

• Fruit such as apples, bananas, grapes, or anything you can cut up and put in a baggie.

• Container of homemade muesli. Combine oats, nuts, flaked coconut, raisins, goji berries, cacao nibs, and so forth. The great thing about this is you can add milk when the flight attendant comes by offering drinks.

• Container or small bag of sugar snap peas for the sweetness and crunch, steamed asparagus, chopped bell pepper, or cucumber and carrot slices.

• Salads in mason jars or sealed containers.

5. Request a meal. Food loses its flavor at high altitudes, so the airline companies pump it full of sugar and salt. Unfortunately, this wreaks havoc on your body. It bloats you, increases water retention, and makes you dehydrated. If you have a long-haul flight, go on the airline's website beforehand and request a vegan, vegetarian, or low-salt meal.

6. Bring mini-packets of spirulina and wheatgrass. Adding these to your water while traveling helps increase energy levels, supply all the essential amino acids, support balanced blood sugar levels, manage cravings, and support mental clarity and focus. Having one packet a day will keep your immune system healthy (especially if you'll be drinking alcohol and eating not-so-healthy foods in your travels).

7. Stock up on magnesium powder or pills to stay regular. One of the worst things about traveling, especially for women, is getting constipated. Avoid this by drinking 8 to 10 cups of water a day, eating fiber-rich foods (think plant-based), and getting your body moving to stimulate your insides. If this isn't effective enough, I always recommend magnesium, which helps to promote using the toilet, not to mention that it helps regulate sleep. If you know that you have a hard time going, try taking some pre-packaged senna tea.

BUT I DON'T EAT ANIMAL PRODUCTS!

Some of the meals I've listed above contain animal products, whether it's feta cheese, honey, or a piece of meat, chicken, or fish. If you're a vegetarian or vegan, don't fret. The after-tox is perfect for you as long as you substitute plant foods wherever necessary. For example, if you find a meal that sounds good, such as the Zucchini Bolognese, but don't eat meat, add tofu or tempeh instead, or chop up some portobello mushrooms. One of my favorite things to do is slice a portobello mushroom and sauté it in coconut oil until it's soft. It has the texture of meat and is a great alternative. If you don't eat honey, use agave syrup, date syrup, or maple syrup. Like the Colorful Crunch Salad but don't want salmon or chicken? Throw on some extra beans or cooked quinoa, or toss it with grilled tofu.

The beautiful thing about clean eating is that there are no strict rules. Simply find what works for you and go with it. Remember, too, that to get maximum results on the after-tox, stick to the three-color rule on your plate, and minimize dairy products, meat, chicken, and fish, as well as any processed foods.

GUIDELINES FOR SUCCESSFUL AFTER-TOXING

By following a few simple guidelines, you'll be able to seamlessly make clean eating a part of your life for infinitely better health. Sound good? Let's review:

1. Fuel your furnace. Eat four to five times a day, three main meals and one or two snacks, in order to keep your body and mind energized while burning calories all day long.

2. Eat at least three plant-based colors in each meal. The more colorful, the more satisfied you feel.

3. Stay hydrated. Drink 2 to 3 liters of water a day, preferably not from a plastic bottle but from a reusable metal or glass bottle. Herbal teas count toward your daily intake.

4. Cut down on coffee and alcohol. If you want to reintroduce them, drink no more than one small cup a day. Opt for red wine instead of other alcoholic drinks, because it contains beneficial antioxidants.

5. Concentrate on eating predominantly alkaline foods (vegetables and fruits). Eat raw foods for lunch, and mostly cooked foods for dinner.

6. Avoid processed and refined foods. These typically come in boxes, jars, or packages; they're low in fiber and high in sugar.

7. Skip packaged foods with health claims on the box. Anything that has to tell you it's healthy means that all the nutrients have been removed and chemicals have been added.

8. Know thy enemies. These include trans fats, fried foods, and added sugar, in all forms.

9. Use your hands as measurements. One snack should be the size of a cupped palm, a full meal no larger than your two hands together, cupped. The stomach is not as big as we think, yet we seem to jam-pack it with as much as possible. Follow these simple rules and you'll never overeat.

10. Choose organic whenever you can.

11. Learn to love certain fats. These are fats that come from vegetable sources, such as nuts, seeds, avocados, and eggs.

12. Eat seasonally and locally. Find out where there are local farmers markets and when produce is delivered into the supermarkets to get it fresh.

13. Get enough sleep to rejuvenate your body, skin, mind, and energy. This will help prevent overeating, beat cravings, promote firm, beautiful skin, and help you lose weight.

14. Plan it so you don't panic. Meal prep is key to clean eating, making the right choices, and improving your willpower.

15. Begin to love yourself—no more self-destruction. Treat yourself the way you treat the people you love. You probably wouldn't talk trash to them, so don't do it to yourself. Being happy in your own mind and body is the most important thing in life.

When you eat clean at least 70 percent of the time, exercise regularly, get enough sleep, and keep going no matter what slip-ups you may have, you'll be on your way to a healthy lifestyle in no time! In fact, you're already there.

CHAPTER 12

DETOX YOUR LIFESTYLE

Over the past two weeks with midterms, I started freaking out, staying up late studying, drinking loads of coffee, and having midnight munchies, which bloated me and set me back so much. I started to feel depressed about my body, so I decided to give your detox a chance. I have gained my confidence back, which to me is the most important. I feel like I'm on top of the world.

—Leidy

Why stop at just cleaning up your body? To really make a truly clean sweep, try to detox your life as well. One of the most important parts of detoxification is how we clear our personal environment, our thoughts, and our emotions. Many of us have toxic habits and feelings that negatively impact our health. These need to be released, too, so that we can truly love ourselves, our bodies, and our lives.

EVERYDAY HOME DETOX

My home is my sanctuary—a place where I can relax and feel safe. I do my best to create a chemical-free environment, with fresh air and peaceful energy in every room.

Over the years, I've learned about how harmful standard household chemicals and cleaning products can be to the body. In the average American household, there are 3 to 10 gallons of hazardous materials and more than sixty hazardous household products! Some of the most prevalent household toxins are sodium hypochlorite, a chemical in chlorine bleach that can irritate the lungs and eyes, and formaldehyde, which is a suspected human carcinogen. Spot removers and carpet cleaners may contain perchloroethylene, another possible cancer-causing agent, and chemicals in disinfectants have been associated with kidney and liver damage.

An alternative to harsh cleaning products is to make your own using white vinegar. Simply combine ½ cup vinegar with ½ gallon water, and fill a spray bottle. It is completely nontoxic and beautifully cleans wood floors, countertops, and kitchen appliances. For a lovely fragrance, add a few drops of mint or lavender essential oil.

You can also make a wonderful natural mosquito repellant by putting ¼ cup lemon juice, 1 tablespoon vanilla extract, and 15 drops lavender oil in a 16-ounce spray bottle and filling the rest of the bottle with water. Mosquitoes hate this stuff. Or you can shop at a health foods store for brands that are formulated without chemicals. Check out the Healthy House Institute at healthyhouseinstitute.com for recommendations of nontoxic products.

I do a lot of cooking, and I prepare food ahead of time for convenience. I prefer to store leftovers in glass containers, rather than plastic. Some plastic containers contain bisphenol A (BPA), a chemical associated with behavioral and neurological problems. If it's more convenient to use plastic containers, stick with those labeled #1, #2, and #4 on the bottom, which signifies they are BPA-free.

The easiest home detox is to vacuum and dust regularly. There are a lot of eco-friendly vacuums on the market that have HEPA filters for extra protection against common allergens. Look for these products in Target and other mass-market retailers.

STRESS DETOX

Our society is overworked, overfed, undernourished, and underexercised. We're constantly under stress from work, school, parents, relationships, or just feeling like we need to respond to everything that comes in on our phones or emails, and all at once. Our levels of stimulation are higher than they've ever been before, and we are no longer taking enough time for ourselves!

We all have our vices. For some it's alcohol, for others it's drugs or cigarettes, and for many it's food. As I mentioned earlier, some people even resort to overexercising, which can become just as obsessive. And it's okay . . . that's human nature.

I get stressed like everyone else, and when I'm stressed, I eat. I hate responding to anxiety with junk food, though. I hate not feeling vibrant and full of energy. I hate waking up with a food hangover the next day. It can be worse than an actual hangover, trust me. I hate how my skin gets dull if I eat poorly, even just one time. On top of all that, stress eating is so bad for your digestive system that, simply put, it forces it to stop working. When all this happens, our bodies are more likely to hold on to every calorie, and morph those calories into love handles that we don't actually love that much.

I share these things because I struggle like everyone else; I've just chosen to be more vocal about it. As I've tried to improve myself and become a better person, I've learned that there are many things I can do to deal more effectively with stress and the negative behaviors it triggers.

My personal stress busters are:

- Regular workouts, whether yoga, weight training, boxing, or walking. Exercise releases feel-good chemicals called endorphins, which quiet anxiety and give you a natural buzz. Working out doesn't have to be time-consuming, either. All it takes for a positive high from exercise is twenty minutes. Nor do you have to sweat your heart out in a gym. Exercising can be as simple as a leisurely hike or playing a sport you love. Moving your body is the key.

- Meditation, coupled with deep breathing. I retreat to a quiet place and feel gratitude for everything I've been given; this definitely reduces my stress levels. According to one study, keeping a gratitude journal and meditating on what you're grateful for decreases stress and depression and boosts happiness. Basically, the practice of gratitude makes negative and anxious feelings evaporate. We can all use a little less negativity and a lot more happiness!

  How often or long should you meditate? Ideally at least for a few minutes every day, but even if you do it once a week, that's better than nothing! Try to start with one minute of deep breathing the moment you wake up, while placing your feet on the ground as you sit on your bed. Close your eyes and breathe in and out, focusing on your breath. Voilà—you have just meditated.

- Smiling. This is the easiest way I've found to lift my spirits instantly, no matter how I'm feeling. And science backs me up. A study published in *Psychological Science* in 2012 showed that smiling during brief periods of anxiety can help to reduce the intensity of the body's stress response (such as rapid heart rate), regardless of whether you actually feel happy. The next time you're stuck in traffic, dealing with a difficult person, or experiencing some other type of stress, hold your face in a smile for a moment—a real genuine, happy smile, not a sarcastic one. (If you need inspiration, think of someone you love or a beautiful place you've been!) Not only will this help calm you down, it might enhance your heart health, too. And it's contagious! When you begin smiling and laughing, those around you tend to do the same. It's a virtuous cycle.

- Positive connections. One of the biggest things I have learned is that I can spend too much time working and too little time with my friends and family. When I was modeling full-time, my workaholism hurt me not only because I got depressed and binge-ate but also because it created tension with my friends and family, who felt like I didn't want to see them. Recently I started making more time to travel to see my family and go out more with my friends, and I've enjoyed every moment of these connections. Life isn't all work and no play. Rather, it is about savoring the experiences we have with others and giving ourselves to the people we love.

- Taking phone and computer breaks. I'll be the first person to tell you how much I love using social media and talking on my phone. These activities have been the catalyst for me to launch some incredible projects and help so many others. But they can also be really draining and make you think your life isn't good enough in comparison to a stranger's seemingly perfect life. People always show the best stuff they've got going and rarely post the bad things. Even knowing that, though, I tend to constantly check my social media accounts and find myself getting hung up on how many likes I get throughout the day! This misguided focus can take away from what's really important.

My solution: Dock your phone in another room at night and don't check it until after breakfast each day. This will help you get all those morning tasks done before getting sucked into that online world. Also, turn it off every once in a while or set a time at night to unplug. Sure, we want to respond to everyone all the time, but this keeps us from being present in our own lives. And please: don't check your phone when you are out with friends, and don't feel you need to share every moment of life on Facebook. With our faces in our devices all the time, life passes us by.

These simple tweaks have helped me enjoy life more and empowered me to battle my own stress demons, instead of just avoiding them. They still pop up from time to time, and probably always will, but at least I know how to deal with them. We may not always be able to control what comes our way, but at least we can control our response with a positive mindset and an open heart.

SLEEP DETOX

I love a good night's sleep. It makes me feel refreshed, restored, and energetic the next day. And that's no accident: sleep allows the body to get rid of toxins and restore itself. If you're suffering from poor-quality sleep, then your body's natural detoxification processes are short-circuited. You may even have trouble controlling your weight, since it'll disrupt the function of your hunger-control hormones. Like most, as I get a busier schedule, I have a harder time sleeping for long hours, but I do make sure to get at least seven to eight hours each night.

Chronic sleep loss also leads to a higher risk of depression, memory problems, headaches, heart palpitations, infections, blood pressure and blood sugar irregularities, and allergic responses such as eczema. As someone who took sleeping pills for years, I can completely relate to anyone who uses them. Sleeping pills and over-the-counter sleep aids are far too common, however. Don't believe the pharmaceutical hype: drugging yourself does not improve sleep quality and will not leave you feeling refreshed! After I began my health journey, I didn't need them anymore. I now understand how to battle the stress that caused those sleepless nights.

If you want healthy sleep, it takes commitment. You really do need to allocate seven to eight hours nightly. So if you get up at 7:30 a.m., put yourself to bed at 11:30 p.m., with at least thirty minutes to read or decompress from the day. I try to follow a pre-sleep routine: I take thirty minutes to wash my face, brush my teeth, and do a little reading—then it's lights out. Within reason, I go to bed and get up at the same time each day.

- Don't bring your cell phone or iPad to bed. This is a biggie—and possibly the worst thing you can do for sleep. These devices expose you to a specific frequency of blue light that messes with levels of the hormone melatonin, delaying sleep and making it harder to stay asleep.
- Use your bedroom only for sleeping and sex—not for watching TV, working on your laptop, or doing projects. Keep your bedroom neat, too—no clutter or mess. Give yourself an extra minute in the morning to make your bed. An organized bedroom supports good sleep and will help declutter your mind.
- Make your bedroom beautiful. Soothing lighting, candles, and nice pillows will immediately bring you peace of mind. If you live in a

place that's noisy or your blinds don't block enough light, use a sleep mask and earplugs, too. These will help you block out all external stimuli so that you can fall asleep faster.

- Exercise, but not too close to bedtime. It increases your body's core temperature, and when you're warm on the inside, you don't sleep as well. It's best to work out several hours prior to bedtime so that your body has time to cool down. When it cools down, you get sleepier.
- Don't eat too close to bedtime, especially starches and sugar. Your blood sugar will rise, and your digestive system will go into overtime trying to digest the food, just when your body is ready to rest.
- Avoid coffee, tea, or other caffeinated beverages late in the evening. A good rule of thumb is to not have any caffeine past 3:00 p.m. If you are very caffeine-sensitive, as I am, cut yourself off at midday, since caffeine can take up to ten hours to exit your system.
- Avoid drinking alcohol after dinner or close to bedtime. As I mentioned earlier, although alcohol is a sedative and might make you feel drowsy, it interferes with the deepest, most restful stages of sleep, leaving you feeling fatigued the next day
- Consider supplementing with "sleep minerals." Calcium and magnesium help promote sleep through their calming action on the nervous system and muscles. Consider taking a calcium and/or magnesium supplement at bedtime; follow the manufacturer's recommendation for dosage.

  Melatonin is another great option, but it can leave some people feeling drowsy the next day. Start with the lowest dose available, and see if this works for you. If it doesn't do the trick, focus on stress reduction and meditation—which are two of the best ways to overcome insomnia naturally.
- Try aromatherapy solutions such as chamomile tea or lavender oil drops on your pillow. Both herbs have sleep-inducing properties, but without the drug-like aftereffects of sleeping pills.
- Visualize something pleasant and serene when the lights go out: a favorite hobby, a creative project, or a destination you like to visit.
- If you're have trouble falling asleep, don't lie there stewing. Instead, get up, leave your bedroom, read a book, and try again a little later.

When I can't sleep, I write down everything I can think of on a piece of paper—every thought, big or small, about what I need to do, what I'm worried about, what's on my mind. This exercise helps get it out of my head and onto paper so I can come back to it in the morning. It helps release things I'm worried about and put me to sleep.

If these strategies don't fix your sleep issues, it's important to consider any underlying causes. They could be hormonal (night sweats), nutritional (insufficient absorption of B vitamins or food irritants in the gut), pharmacological (stimulants), physiological (sleep apnea), and/or psychological (stress). Seek help from your doctor, a provider of natural healthcare, or a mental health therapist to help you pinpoint the problem and alleviate your insomnia so that sleep restoration may begin.

EMOTIONAL DETOX

We all know that having emotional issues can lead to problems with food: overeating, bingeing, and for some people starvation. We use food to celebrate and to combat fear and anxiety. But as with alcohol or any other crutch, it's the underlying emotion that must be detoxed and resolved—otherwise it can erode your vitality, self-image, and sense of personal value. It can also trigger physical symptoms such as chronic back pain, migraines, fatigue, sleep problems, and poor immunity. Whether you're struggling with your weight, health, job, or relationships, you may have stored-up toxic feelings that make you feel sluggish and dull. I know that after I do an emotional detox, I feel revitalized. All the energy I was using to suppress pain and sweep emotional issues under the carpet becomes available for more creative, positive pursuits.

- Understand the binge response. A lot of people struggle with bingeing at one time or another, typically when they have an emotional issue and use food to self-medicate or self-soothe rather than dealing directly with the problem. And the binge only makes them feel worse. It's a vicious cycle. Changing that behavior is tough because it becomes so habitual. There are no easy answers, but the bottom line is that you have to develop a new relationship with food, in which it is not an emotional fallback but a source of fuel. Try to:

- Eat only when you're physically hungry.
- Eat mindfully and joyfully, not while watching TV or doing something else.
- Learn about the wonderful nutrients in clean food and imagine them working inside you on your behalf.
- Visualize yourself as someone who is strong, not dependent on food to de-stress.
- Don't beat yourself up if you have a binge.
- Keep a sense of humor. The next time you want to dive into a gallon of ice cream, imagine it sitting on your hips. Not so attractive now, is it?

Don't give up, even if you seem to keep trying and failing. You *can* change. It's not luck or magic. It's perseverance and the desire to stop self-destructive habits. After a few months of paying attention to your behavior, your relationship to food—and whatever else might be getting you down—will improve.

- Figure out what's bugging you. Why are you down? Why are you anxious? Why are you lashing out? Emotions like depression, anger, or frustration often stem from specific events, such as a breakup or divorce, the death of a loved one, financial problems, or a layoff. For others, they stem from a sense that you should be doing more with your life. Answering these questions honestly helps you identify the source of your negativity.

It always helps me to find a quiet space—no TV, no conversations, no computer or cell phone—in which I can contemplate my issues and bring them into more conscious awareness. Then I can deal with them more mindfully and start to problem solve. Once you've identified the source of your negative emotions, you've taken the first step toward resolution and are better equipped to take action. Say you've just gone through a breakup. As tough as it can be to take that first step, make an effort one night this week to meet new people, head to a new workout class, or do something else positive for yourself: plan a vacation or a makeover or another brand-new experience.

Action is the perfect antidote to most of the things that make us sad, depressed, or emotionally paralyzed. Whatever you do, don't ignore the underlying emotions. One of my favorite quotes is, "Just when the caterpillar thought the world was over, it became a butterfly." All good things take time, hard work, and persistence, even when the night seems darkest.

· Consider an emotional cleansing ritual. Once you know what's been eating away at you—anger at a friend, a resentment or grudge you've been holding on to, a frustration you've been bearing—create a ritual to release it: throw a stone into the water, write a letter and burn it or tear it up, visualize its dissipation into the air, or whatever else helps you consciously let go of the toxic emotions holding you hostage. This simple act can be very powerful and help free you emotionally. Unless you let these things go, you'll erode your sense of vitality, self-esteem, and worth. Trust me on this.

· Seek expert help. If you feel depressed or hopeless for more than two weeks, seek support from a professional psychologist or counselor. Some issues do require a higher level of intervention, and there is nothing wrong with asking for it.

It's easy to cruise through life, ignoring the issues that might be lurking underneath your physical or mental distress, and then all of a sudden, it's not so simple anymore, and you feel stuck and bleak. Let's break the cycle together. If bad things happen—and they will—you'll want the strength to not beat yourself up but to respond positively and move forward. Cleansing yourself physically and emotionally builds that strength. You'll find that your whole outlook on life will change—because you're correctly feeding your body *and* your soul.

FINAL NOTE

Just remember, all it takes is one decision to make a change, no matter how big or small. The key is to think about where you are and where you want to go. What motivates you to change? There are no right or wrong reasons to get healthier, lose weight, or detoxify your body and mind; the key is to make sure you are doing it for yourself.

One of the biggest things I want you to take away from doing the detox is that no matter how far you have to go, or whether you are already at a place you love, this detox will help to create a better you. Because no two days are the same in life, this means that each time you do it, you have the power to learn more about nutrition, what works for your body, and how to clear blockages in your mind. I want you to know that you can do this. It's five days that will change the way you look at life, and the positive aftereffects will lead you into a journey that is filled with beautiful food for permanent weight control. If you are struggling during the five days, do your best and try it once again next month, seeing if you can stick to it even more.

Like all people in life, there have been times I've done the detox and cheated on it, while other times it was smooth sailing. I want you to remember that even if you cannot do the detox 100 percent as written, that's okay. The wonderful thing about life is that with each new day, you have a choice to become healthier and happier. Perfection is not the goal here; heck, there is no such thing as perfection, since we all have flaws in our lives. The goal is to be better than you were yesterday. Whether that means swapping over from milk in your latte to soy milk or cutting down on cigarettes, each positive choice you make will lead you one step closer to becoming the person you want to be.

Think about your health journey as bridges. Before you can get to each new place, you must cross a bridge. For me, that was starting off with soy milk in my coffee, then moving on to premade almond milk, and now I'm making my own nut milks. The same goes for moving from eating conventional meat products to organic ones to now eating organic meat only occasionally. It's all about making small steps so you know they will stick, and enjoying the process as you go along.

Just like everyone else, I was not born a good cook, nor did I love fruits or vegetables. I didn't thrive on exercise, and I didn't care about meditation. I was your everyday person (and still am, really!) who loved takeout, fast-food joints, having wine or cocktails with friends, and fitting in with the crowd. Now I realize that I can still do these things, just in moderation, backed by a healthier way of eating and a more balanced, peaceful lifestyle. I also love fitting *out* of the crowd, because I'm proud to be unique and my own person, without following what other people say and do. All of this has led me to a far greater place of happiness and gratitude, and it's something that I am passionate about sharing with others.

Whether you are still struggling to make a change or have loved every moment of the detox and the recipes afterward, I invite you to head over to my website, nikkisharp.com, where you can find many resources: more recipes and guides to meditation, healthier living, and exercising.

As always, thank you so much for reading this book. I hope that it's inspired you to make a change in your life and to become a happier and healthier person, both for yourself and for those around you.

With love, Nikki

ACKNOWLEDGMENTS

As I write this, there are so many people to whom I wish I could specifically say thank you. I have met countless individuals who have given me inspiration and helped me to be present, be grateful, and become a model-turned-author with a book that is changing the world. To those of you who are not mentioned and were a part of this book—thank you, thank you, thank you. I am forever grateful for your help whether directly or indirectly on making this book what it is.

Mom and Dad, I am grateful for the lessons you have taught me, the ones I learned from watching, and those from doing. You both have allowed me to be a free bird and learn about life in my own ways, while giving me advice and being there when I needed it most. Jim, thank you for being in my life. You've taught me what it means to have dedication, no matter what happens, and an invaluable lesson on how to treat people.

Thank you so much to the whole team who worked on the beautiful photos for this book, including Ray Kachatorian, Jennifer Barguiarena,

Vivian Lui, Kelly Shew, Toven Stith, and many others. You helped to put my vision into the pages here, and I am so grateful. To my book agents, Steve Troha and Scott Hoffman, thank you both for being here with me during the whole process of writing this book. After all the meetings, emails, calls, and time spent on everything from the proposal to the manuscript, it's finally here! To everyone at Ballantine, a huge thank-you for believing in my vision and working on making this book so beautiful. Specifically: Jennifer Tun, Richard Callison, Nina Shield, Ted Allen, Liz Cosgrove, Joseph Perez, Mark Maguire, and Jenn Backe, thank you for your time, dedication, and hard work. I am so grateful to each one of you.

Namrata, Samantha, Gina, Sara, Ashlee, and Steven and Kirsten, thank you for sharing your "before" and "after" photo to be used in this book (and thanks to those who gave permission, although we didn't use your photo). I hope it helps you find continued success in your health journey! Surachai Saengsuwan, Jon Attenborough, and Sasha Rainbow: I'm so happy to be able to include the modeling photos you took, so without sounding like a broken record, a big thanks to you three as well.

And finally, to Bianca, the woman who shared her innermost secrets with me and asked for my advice when I had just started my Instagram account: Thank you. You don't know this, but you forever changed the course of my life, because after this I realized it was my life's mission to help people and to make a difference in the world of health. Wherever you are, you have been in my mind since your first email, and I graciously thank you.

APPENDIX A: YOUR 5-DAY JOURNAL

DAY _____

Breakfast: _____
_____
_____
_____

Snack #1: _____
_____
_____
_____

Lunch: _____
_____
_____
_____

Snack #2: _____
_____
_____
_____

Dinner: _____
_____
_____
_____

Water servings: _____

Starting weight (Day 1): _____

Ending weight (Day 6): _____

TODAY'S ACTIVITIES AND THOUGHTS

Physical Activity (if any)

Description: _____
_____
_____
_____

Duration: _____

My Energy Level

Morning:
• High   • Moderate   • Low

Afternoon:
• High   • Moderate   • Low

Evening:
• High   • Moderate   • Low

My Emotions

Morning: _____
_____
_____

Evening: _____
_____
_____

Symptoms (if any): _____
_____
_____

Today I am grateful for: _____
_____
_____
_____

APPENDIX B
THE SHARP LIFETIME DIET RECIPES

BREAKFAST RECIPES

TOMATO BOMBS

(SERVES 1–2)

Ingredients:

2 fresh tomatoes
2 medium organic eggs
1 slice gluten-free bread

Sea salt
Black pepper
1 green onion, chopped

Directions:

1. Preheat the oven to 350 degrees F.

2. Cut off the tops of the tomatoes, remove the seeds, and scoop out the insides, leaving a big enough gap for the egg.

3. Crack 1 egg into each tomato. Place the filled tomatoes on a baking pan and bake for 5 minutes, or until egg is solid.

4. Toast the bread and cut into strips.

5. Remove the tomatoes from the oven. Sprinkle them with salt, pepper, and chopped green onion, and serve with the toast.

Tip: A drop of Worcestershire sauce or sprinkle of cayenne pepper is a lovely addition.

SUPERFOOD SMOOTHIE

(SERVES 1)

Ingredients:

1 banana
½ cup blueberries
½ cup strawberries
1 tablespoon acai powder

¼ teaspoon cinnamon
2 pitted Medjool dates
⅛ teaspoon organic vanilla extract
   (optional)

Directions:

Place all ingredients in a blender and add 1 cup ice. Blend until smooth.

LEAN CLEAN OATMEAL

(SERVES 1)

Ingredients:

¼ medium zucchini, grated
¼ cup oats
2 egg whites
½ teaspoon vanilla extract

Stevia
Fresh fruit, goji berries, cacao nibs,
   or cinnamon for topping (optional)

Directions:

1. In a pot over medium heat, combine the zucchini, oats, egg whites, and ¼ cup water. Stir until the oats have cooked and egg whites have mixed in and solidified, roughly 5 minutes.

2. Add the vanilla and stevia to taste.

3. Serve topped with fresh fruit, goji berries, cacao nibs, cinnamon, or anything else you desire.

HIGH-PROTEIN PANCAKES

(SERVES 1)

Ingredients:

1 ripe banana, mashed
2 eggs, beaten
1 tablespoon coconut oil

Fresh berries, yogurt, cinnamon,
   or chopped mint for topping
   (optional)

Directions:

1. Mix the banana with the eggs until smooth.

2. In a medium skillet, melt the coconut oil over medium-low heat. Ladle the banana batter into the pan. Cook the pancakes about 2 to 3 minutes on each side.

3. If desired, top with fresh berries (try goji berries) and 1 tablespoon Greek yogurt or coconut yogurt. Sprinkle with cinnamon or top with chopped mint (my favorite).

VERY BERRY SMOOTHIE

(SERVES 1)

Ingredients:

1 banana, frozen
2 cups mixed berries
1 handful spinach

Squeeze of lime
¼ teaspoon vanilla extract
1 handful mint

Directions:

Place all ingredients in a blender with 1 cup water. Blend until smooth.

GINGER SMOOTHIE

(SERVES 1)

Ingredients:

3 carrots, grated
1 apple, chopped
1 cucumber, chopped

½ lemon, peel and pith removed, sliced
1-inch piece ginger, peeled and
   chopped

Directions:

Place all ingredients in a blender or food processor, along with a handful of ice. Blend until smooth.

SHARPIES SOS SMOOTHIE

(SERVES 1)

Ingredients:

¼ avocado, peeled and chopped
½ cucumber, chopped
Juice of ½ lime
1 handful spinach

1 handful kale
1 teaspoon spirulina
1 apple, cored and chopped

Directions:

Place all ingredients in a blender or food processor. Blend until smooth.

LUNCH RECIPES

SPRING FORWARD SALAD

(SERVES 1)

Ingredients:

1 tablespoon coconut oil
½ eggplant, diced into cubes
2 cups mixed spinach and arugula
¼ cup kidney beans, rinsed and
    drained
½ avocado, peeled and sliced
½ can hearts of palm, rinsed, drained,
    and chopped
1 large carrot, peeled and chopped

2 tablespoons sprouted lentils
1 tablespoon olive oil
1 tablespoon tahini
1 tablespoon fresh lime juice
2 tablespoons fresh orange juice
Sea salt
Cayenne pepper
Cracked black pepper

Directions:

1. In a skillet, heat the coconut oil over medium heat and add the eggplant. Cook for 5 minutes, or until lightly browned and soft. Transfer to a bowl.

2. Add the spinach, arugula, kidney beans, avocado, hearts of palm, carrot, and lentils to the eggplant and mix.

3. To make the dressing, whisk together the oil, tahini, lime juice, and orange juice. Season with salt, cayenne, and black pepper. Toss with the salad.

GARDEN SALAD

(SERVES 1)

Ingredients:

1 tablespoon pine nuts
1 cup mixed salad greens
¼ cup cooked chickpeas
1 cup fresh raspberries
¼ cup feta cheese

2 tablespoons apple cider vinegar
2 tablespoons balsamic vinegar
2 teaspoons honey
1 tablespoon Dijon mustard
2 tablespoons olive oil

Directions:

1. Gently toast the pine nuts in a 300-degree F oven and set aside to cool.

2. Place the salad greens, chickpeas, and ½ cup raspberries in a large bowl.

3. Cut the feta into small chunks and sprinkle over the salad and berries. Add the pine nuts.

4. To make the dressing, combine the remaining ½ cup raspberries, both vinegars, honey, and mustard in a blender or food processor and puree until smooth. With the motor running, slowly pour in the oil and blend until well combined.

ZUCCHINI PASTA SALAD

(SERVES 1)

Ingredients:

½ yellow summer squash
½ zucchini
¼ avocado, peeled and chopped
¼ head purple cabbage, chopped
1 large carrot (or 3 small), peeled
   and chopped
3 radishes, chopped
¼ cup mixed berries

Small handful basil, chopped
2 tablespoons olive oil
Juice of 1 lemon
1 tablespoon mustard
1 tablespoon agave or honey
⅛ teaspoon cayenne pepper
⅛ teaspoon turmeric

Directions:

1. Use a spiralizer or vegetable peeler to turn the summer squash and zucchini into "noodles." Place in a salad bowl.

2. Add avocado, cabbage, carrots, radishes, and berries to the "noodles."

3. Prepare the dressing by whisking the remaining ingredients together.

4. Toss the salad with the dressing. Place in the refrigerator for 10 minutes to allow the vegetables to soften.

HUMMUS WRAP

(SERVES 1)

Ingredients:

One 16-ounce can garbanzo beans
   (chickpeas), drained and rinsed
Juice of 1 lemon
1 tablespoon tahini
1 tablespoon olive oil
1 medium carrot, peeled and chopped
Sea salt

Black pepper
1 sandwich wrap
½ cucumber, sliced lengthwise
¼ cabbage, sliced
1 large carrot, shredded
½ avocado, sliced

Directions:

1. Combine the chickpeas, lemon juice, tahini, oil, and chopped carrot in a blender or food processor. Season with salt and pepper. Blend until well combined. Add a dash of water if needed, or an extra teaspoon of olive oil.

2. Lay the wrap in front of you. Spread the hummus on the wrap, leaving about 1 inch on the far edge empty. Add the cucumber, cabbage, shredded carrot, and avocado.

3. Start rolling with the side nearest you. Cut the rolled wrap in half.

HOMEMADE BURGERS WITH CARAMELIZED ONIONS

(2 SERVINGS)

Ingredients:

8 ounces 90 percent lean ground beef
   (or use buffalo or turkey for less fat)
1 small handful arugula, finely chopped
Sea salt
Black pepper
Cayenne pepper

1 medium onion, chopped
1 to 2 tablespoons honey
Whole-grain buns or large iceberg
   lettuce leaves
Tomato or avocado slices

Directions:

1. In a bowl, combine the meat and arugula. Add salt, pepper, and cayenne to taste. Mix well and form into two patties, or four if you want thin ones.

2. Place the patties in a nonstick skillet and cook on medium heat for 5 minutes. Flip and cook another 5 minutes.

3. In a separate skillet, combine the onions and 2 tablespoons water. Cook on medium heat until onions are tender. Drain off any excess water. Add the

honey and cook another few minutes until all the onions are very soft and slightly sticky.

4. If you are serving the patties on buns, toast them in the oven. Otherwise, use lettuce leaves. Place a bun half or lettuce leaf on a plate, add a patty, then layer with tomato and avocado. Top with the caramelized onions.

ASIAN SPRING ROLLS

(SERVES 1)

Ingredients:

One 15-ounce can chickpeas, drained and rinsed
1 handful cilantro
Sea salt
Black pepper
1 tablespoon tahini
1 tablespoon olive oil
½ cup raw beets, grated
2 brown rice wrappers

3 ounces of shredded chicken
1 handful of a mixture of alfalfa sprouts, chopped cilantro, and chopped kale
½ avocado, peeled and chopped
Liquid aminos
Cider vinegar
Balsamic vinegar

Directions:

1. To make the hummus, combine the chickpeas, cilantro, salt and pepper to taste, tahini, oil, and beets in a blender or food processor with a dash of water. Blend well.

2. Soak the rice wrappers in hot water for 20 seconds, until soft. Place them on a cutting board. On half of each wrapper spread some of the hummus and then top with the chicken, greens mixture, and avocado. Starting with the side that has the hummus, fold the wrapper over like a burrito, turning in the sides as you roll. Cut the rolls in half.

3. Make a dipping sauce by combining the liquid aminos and vinegars to taste. Serve the sauce with the rolls.

CAULIFLOWER PIZZA

(SERVES 1–3)

Ingredients:

½ head cauliflower, chopped
2 tablespoons almond meal (ground almonds)
1 teaspoon oregano
1 egg
1 large tomato
1 small squeeze tomato paste (optional)

1 small head garlic, cloves separated and peeled
1 handful basil
Olive oil
Cracked black pepper
Cayenne pepper (optional)
Chopped artichoke hearts, chopped zucchini, sliced red bell pepper, and sliced mushrooms, for topping
1 handful spinach, for topping

Directions:

1. Preheat the oven to 350 degrees F.

2. Pulse the cauliflower in a blender or food processor to create a "rice" (it should be quite fine). Place in a bowl and microwave 5 minutes, or place in a pan and cook over medium-high heat until soft. When cool, place the cauliflower in a clean kitchen towel and squeeze out all excess liquid. (The more liquid you get out, the better the crust will stay together when you cook it.)

3. With your hands, mix the cauliflower, almond meal, oregano, and egg in a bowl until well combined. Pat the mixture about ¼ inch thick onto a cookie sheet lined with parchment paper. Bake for 20 minutes, or until lightly browned.

4. While the crust is baking, prepare the sauce. Combine the tomato, tomato paste (if using), garlic, basil, and a drizzle of olive oil in a blender or food processor and blend until smooth. Season with black pepper and cayenne. Pour the sauce into a small pot and cook over medium heat until heated through.

5. Spread the sauce over the baked crust.

6. Place the artichoke hearts, zucchini, red pepper, and mushrooms in a small pot with a little water. Cook for 2 minutes over medium heat until the vegetables are slightly tender. Top the pizza with these veggies, along with the spinach. Place the pizza back in the oven for 5 minutes. Let cool for a few minutes prior to serving.

MEDITERRANEAN LASAGNA

(SERVES 1)

Ingredients:

1 zucchini, cut lengthwise into long, thin strips

Sea salt

One 15-ounce can organic crushed tomatoes (look for a brand without added sugar)

4 sun-dried tomatoes, or to taste

10 basil leaves, chopped

1 clove garlic

1 to 2 tablespoons olive oil

Cayenne pepper

1 tablespoon chia seeds

1 to 2 tablespoons crumbled feta cheese

Cracked black pepper

Toasted pine nuts (optional)

Directions:

1. Sprinkle the zucchini with salt and let sit for 20 minutes. Rinse off the salt and squeeze out the excess moisture.

2. Combine the crushed tomatoes, sun-dried tomatoes, 7 of the basil leaves, garlic, and oil in a blender or food processor. Season with cayenne and salt. Blend until completely smooth, or leave it a bit chunky if that's your preference.

3. Add the sauce to a pan, along with the chia seeds, and heat for 1 to 2 minutes.

4. Begin layering in a small glass baking dish, starting with 2 strips of the zucchini on the bottom. Spoon the sauce over the zucchini, add a few crumbles of cheese, and top with another layer of zucchini. Repeat the layering process until all is gone. Top with remaining basil, cracked pepper, and toasted pine nuts (optional).

CABBAGE PATCH WRAPS

(SERVES 1)

Ingredients:

¼ cup uncooked quinoa

2 tablespoons cider vinegar

Chopped cilantro

Cayenne

1 small chicken breast

¼ zucchini, chopped

1 medium tomato, chopped

1 large carrot, half of it chopped and the other half julienned

1 red bell pepper, half of it chopped and the other half julienned

2 tablespoons olive oil

1 tablespoon balsamic vinegar

1 teaspoon turmeric

4 leaves of a red or green cabbage, peeled off

¼ pack snap peas, julienned

Chopped basil

Directions:

1. In a pot, combine the quinoa and ¾ cup water. Bring the quinoa to a boil, reduce the heat to low, cover, and cook for 10 to 15 minutes, or until the quinoa has absorbed all the liquid and is tender. Stir in 1 tablespoon cider vinegar, chopped cilantro to taste, and a pinch of cayenne, and set aside.

2. In another pot cover the chicken with water. Cook, covered, over medium heat for 15 minutes, until all the pink is gone from the center of the chicken breast. Shred or chop the cooked chicken.

3. In a blender or food processor, pulse the zucchini, tomato, chopped carrot, chopped bell pepper, oil, balsamic vinegar, the remaining 1 tablespoon cider vinegar, 1 teaspoon cayenne, and 1 teaspoon turmeric to make a salsa. Set aside.

4. In a pan bring about an inch of water to a boil and add one of the cabbage leaves. Cook for about 2 minutes, until softened. Remove and let cool. Repeat the process with the next leaf.

5. Lay a leaf in front of you. Add a thin layer of the quinoa, then top with the julienned carrot, bell pepper, and snap peas. Add chopped basil to taste, some shredded chicken, and some sauce. Fold both ends toward the center, grab the side of the cabbage leaf closest to you and fold over, making sure all the ingredients stay inside. Fold it like a burrito.

ZUCCHINI BOLOGNESE

(1 LARGE OR 2 SMALL SERVINGS)

Ingredients:

1 large zucchini
4 ounces of 95 percent lean
    shredded beef
Cayenne pepper
Cracked black pepper
1 clove garlic, crushed
Small handful cherry tomatoes

1 tablespoon olive oil
Fresh basil
Dried oregano
Sea salt (optional)
Nutritional yeast or shredded
    Parmesan

Directions:

1. Cut the ends off the zucchini. If you have a spiralizer, use any of the settings to create the noodles. Otherwise, use a vegetable peeler to create zucchini "noodles."

2. Bring 2 cups of water to a boil and add the zucchini. Cook for about 2 minutes, or until tender. Drain and set aside.

3. Cook the beef in a pan over medium heat, breaking it up, until it is no longer pink. Season with cayenne and black pepper.

4. In a small skillet, combine the garlic, cherry tomatoes, and oil and cook over

medium heat until the tomatoes burst. Season with cayenne, black pepper, basil, and oregano. (For a quicker if slightly less tasty version, you can blend those ingredients in a blender or food processor.)

5. Add the tomato mixture to the cooked beef, stir, and add salt to taste.

6. Add the zucchini noodles to the pan and heat through.

7. Plate the Bolognese and sprinkle with nutritional yeast, which adds a cheesy flavor without additional calories, salt, or fat. Another option is to use a little bit of shredded Parmesan cheese.

MOROCCAN DINNER SALAD
(SERVES 1)

Ingredients:

1 cup mixed red and orange cherry tomatoes, halved
¼ cup cooked chickpeas, rinsed and drained
¼ cup chopped cucumber
¼ cup crumbled feta cheese
¼ cup cooked quinoa

1 handful chopped mint
1 handful chopped parsley
Fresh lemon juice
Olive oil
Sea salt
Black pepper

Directions:

In a large bowl, mix the tomatoes, chickpeas, cucumber, cheese, quinoa, mint, and parsley. Drizzle with lemon juice and olive oil and season with salt and pepper.

CHANA MASALA
(SERVES 1)

Ingredients:

1 tablespoon olive oil
½ medium onion, thinly sliced
One 3-inch piece ginger, peeled and thinly sliced
3 cloves garlic, minced
2 green chiles, finely chopped
1 teaspoon mustard seeds
½ teaspoon cumin seeds
One 15-ounce can plum tomatoes
1½ teaspoons turmeric

One 15-ounce can chickpeas, drained and rinsed
½ teaspoon sea salt
½ teaspoon black pepper
2 handfuls cilantro
1 fresh tomato, diced
¼ large avocado, diced
Squeeze of lemon
Drizzle of balsamic vinegar
1 large romaine lettuce leaf

Directions:

1. In a small skillet, heat the oil over medium heat. Add the onion and ginger and sauté for 3 minutes. Add the garlic, chiles, mustard seeds, and cumin. Sauté until the vegetables are softened and lightly browned.

2. Add the tomatoes and turmeric and simmer for 10 minutes, adding water if necessary. Add the chickpeas and cook for another 5 minutes, adding water if necessary. Season with salt and pepper and garnish with about two-thirds of the cilantro.

3. To make the salad, mix the fresh tomato, avocado, lemon juice, balsamic vinegar, and remaining cilantro and place on a lettuce leaf.

Tip: This dish can be served with Greek yogurt, quinoa, brown rice, or any other accompaniments you may wish to have.

SNACKS

KILLER KALE SMOOTHIE

(SERVES 1)

Ingredients:

1 cup unsweetened almond milk
1 tablespoon almond butter
1 banana, frozen
3 dates, pitted

2 cups kale
½ cup broccoli, chopped
1 tablespoon hemp seeds

Directions:

Place all ingredients in a blender and blend until smooth.

PIÑA COLADA SMOOTHIE

(SERVES 1)

Ingredients:

½ cup unsweetened almond milk
½ cup coconut water
½ cup pineapple chunks

1 teaspoon honey
1 tablespoon shredded coconut
¼ teaspoon vanilla

Directions:

Place all ingredients, along with ice, in a blender and blend until smooth.

JUNGLE JUICE

(SERVES 1)

Ingredients:

1 handful spinach
1 handful lettuce
2 celery stalks

¼ fresh pineapple, peeled and cored
½ lime, peeled

Directions:

Run all ingredients through a juicer, according to the manufacturer's instructions.

UP BEET

(SERVES 1)

Ingredients:

1 apple
1 beet
1 cup broccoli
½ celery stalk
¼ cucumber

¼-inch piece fresh ginger
1 handful kale
Juice of ¼ lemon
1 handful parsley

Directions:

Run all ingredients through a juicer, according to the manufacturer's instructions.

BLISS BALLS

(SERVES 1)

Ingredients:

1 cup raw almonds
1 cup pitted Medjool dates
1 tablespoon orange zest
1 tablespoon orange juice
1 teaspoon lemon juice
½ teaspoon turmeric

¼ teaspoon sea salt
½ teaspoon maca powder
¼ cup coconut flakes (or dried shred-
    ded coconut)

Directions:

1. In a food processor or blender, start by processing the almonds and dates until well combined. Add ½ tablespoon orange zest, orange juice, lemon juice, turmeric, salt, and maca powder. Process until smooth. Transfer the mixture to a bowl.

2. Roll the mixture into one-inch balls.

3. If using coconut flakes, process in the food processor until they're in small pieces. Alternatively, use desiccated coconut. Add the remaining ½ tablespoon of orange zest and mix.

4. Coat the balls in the coconut mixture. Place on a baking sheet and freeze for 30 minutes.

DESSERTS

RAW CARROT CUPCAKES

(SERVES 1)

Ingredients:

3 large carrots, peeled and chopped
6 Medjool dates
1 teaspoon coconut oil
1 tablespoon chia seeds (optional)
1 tablespoon coconut flakes
1 teaspoon cinnamon

1 teaspoon pumpkin pie spice or nutmeg
½ cup chopped walnuts
¼ cup coconut butter, melted
Maple syrup
½ teaspoon turmeric

Directions:

1. To make the cakes, combine the carrots, dates, coconut oil, chia seeds (if using), coconut, cinnamon, and pumpkin pie spice in food processor. Process until well combined (or leave the carrots a little chunkier—your choice).

2. Transfer the carrot mixture to a bowl and fold in the walnuts.

3. Fill mini cupcake papers with the carrot mixture. Place a holder in your hand to hold its shape as you fill it using a spoon.

4. To prepare the frosting, blend the coconut butter, 1 tablespoon maple syrup or to taste, and turmeric in a blender or food processor until smooth. You might need to add some water to get it creamier; start with 1 tablespoon and add more as needed.

5. Place the frosting in a zip-top bag. Cut a small hole in one corner and pipe the frosting onto the tops of the cakes. Freeze the frosted cupcakes for 20 minutes before serving. Store in the freezer or refrigerator.

GREEN TEA ICE CREAM

(SERVES 1)

Ingredients:

2 ripe bananas, peeled and frozen
1 small handful mint
1 teaspoon matcha green tea powder
¼ cup coconut milk (optional)
1 tablespoon honey or agave syrup
 (optional)

Toppings: Sliced almonds, additional chopped mint, or cacao nibs for topping

Directions:

1. Place all ingredients into a blender or food processor and blend until smooth and creamy. At this point, your mixture will resemble soft serve, and it's totally delectable. If you'd like it harder, place it in a bowl and freeze for 30 minutes.

2. Top with sliced almonds, chopped mint, or my favorite, cacao nibs.

TRIPLE-LAYER BERRY CHEESECAKE

(SERVES 1)

Ingredients:

½ cup nuts or seeds (walnuts, almonds, Brazil nuts, or pumpkin seeds)
½ cup pitted Medjool dates
Sea salt
1 small handful coconut flakes (optional)
1½ cups cashews, soaked in water for at least 4 hours and drained

Juice of 1–2 lemons
1–2 teaspoons vanilla extract
¼ cup virgin coconut oil
⅓ cup honey or agave syrup
1 cup strawberries, blueberries, or raspberries
Cacao nibs, goji berries, or additional berries for topping

Directions:

1. In a food processor, combine the nuts or seeds, dates, a pinch of salt, and the coconut (if using) and pulse until a dough forms. Press the dough into the bottom of a springform pan.

2. Combine the soaked cashews, lemon juice, vanilla, coconut oil, and honey. Blend until completely smooth, scraping down the sides as necessary.

3. Pour ⅔ of the cashew mixture over the crust, smoothing over with a spoon. To the remaining ⅓ of the cashew mixture, add the berries and blend until smooth. Pour over the first layer.

4. Top the mixture with cacao nibs, goji berries, or extra berries and place in the freezer for 2 hours. Remove and semi-thaw before serving, or eat frozen.

RAW CHOCOLATE MOUSSE TARTS

(5 SERVINGS)

Ingredients:

½ cup almonds
½ cup pitted dates
1 tablespoon chia seeds
Sea salt
Cayenne pepper

½ banana
½ avocado
2 tablespoons raw cacao powder
1 tablespoon maple syrup or agave
1 teaspoon vanilla extract

Directions:

1. Combine the almonds, dates, chia seeds, a pinch of salt, and a pinch of cayenne in a food processor or blender and pulse until the crust ingredients form a sticky dough.

2. Divide the dough into 5 pieces. Press each piece into the bottom and up the sides of a silicone cupcake liner. Place in the freezer for 30 minutes.

3. Combine the banana, avocado, cacao powder, maple syrup, and vanilla in a food processor or blender and process until smooth. Divide the mixture among the crusts.

4. Place the tarts back in the freezer for another 20 minutes. Then remove them from the liners.

APPENDIX C
REFERENCES

CHAPTER 1: DETOXING WITH CLEAN FOOD

Bornman, R., et al. 2010. DDT and urogenital malformations in newborn boys in a malarial area. *BJUI Journal* 106: 405–411.

Environmental Working Group. 2005. Body burden: the pollution in newborns. Online: www.ewg.org, July 14.

Giesecke, K., et al. 1989. Protein and amino acid metabolism during early starvation as reflected by excretion of urea and methylhistidines. *Metabolism* 38: 1196–1200.

Hamilton, A.S., and Mack, T.M. 2003. Puberty and genetic susceptibility to breast cancer in a case-control study in twins. *New England Journal of Medicine* 348: 2313–2322.

Joseph, J., et al. 2009. Nutrition, brain aging, and neurogeneration. *Journal of Neuroscience* 29: 12795–127801.

Klein, A.V., and Kiat, H. 2014. Detox diets for toxin elimination and weight management: a critical review of the evidence. *Journal of Human Nutrition and Dietetics*, December 18, 1–10.

Oliver, L.C., and Shackleton, B.W. 1998. The indoor air we breathe. *Public Health Reports* 113: 398–409.

Wojciciki, J.M., and Heyman, M.B. 2012. Reducing childhood obesity by eliminating 100% fruit juice. *American Journal of Public Health* 102: 1630–1633.

CHAPTER 2: WHY IT WORKS: THE METABOLIC DETOX PRINCIPLES

De la Casa Almeida, M., et al. 2013. Cellulite's aetiology: a review. *European Academy of Dermatology and Venereology* 27: 273–278.

Kapusta-Duch, J., et al. 2012. The beneficial effects of Brassica vegetables on human health. *Roczniki Państwowego Zakładu Higieny* 63: 389–395.

McKnight, W. 2013. Vegetarian, vegan diets yield significant weight loss. *Family Practice News*, December 1.

Schwalfenberg, G. 2012. The alkaline diet: is there evidence that an alkaline pH diet benefits health? *Journal of Environmental and Public Health* Epub, October 12.

CHAPTER 3: WHAT TO EAT: FOODS THAT CLEANSE AND PEEL OFF POUNDS

Hursel, R., and Westerterp-Plantenga. 2010. Thermogenic ingredients and body weight regulation. *International Journal of Obesity* 34: 659–669.

CHAPTER 5: THE PRE-TOX

Baranski, M., et al. 2014. Higher antioxidant and lower cadmium concentrations and lower incidence of pesticide residues in organically grown crops: a systematic literature review and meta-analyses. *British Journal of Nutrition* 112: 794–811.

CHAPTER 6: THE 5-DAY PLAN

Canoy, D., et al. 2005. Plasma ascorbic acid concentrations and fat distribution in 19,068 British men and women in the European Prospective Investigation into Cancer and Nutrition Norfolk cohort study. *American Journal of Clinical Nutrition* 82: 1203–1209.

Mizoguchi, T., et al. 2008. Nutrigenomic studies of effects of Chlorella on subjects with high-risk factors for lifestyle-related disease. *Journal of Medicinal Food* 11: 395–404.

Zemel, M.B. 2003. Mechanisms of dairy modulation of adiposity. *Journal of Nutrition* 133: 252S–256S.

CHAPTER 7: THE GUY-TOX: CALLING ALL MEN

Despres, P. 2011. Excess visceral adipose tissue/ectopic fat the missing link in the obesity paradox? *Journal of the American College of Cardiology* 57: 1887–1889.

Hairston, K.G., et al. 2012. Lifestyle factors and 5-year abdominal fat accumulation in a minority cohort: the IRAS Family Study. *Obesity* 20: 421–427.

Nikolic, D., et al. 2004. Metabolism of 8-prenylnaringenin, a potent phytoestrogen from hops (Humulus lupulus), by human liver microsomes. *Drug Metabolism and Disposition* 32: 272–279.

Tsai, S.A., et al. 2015. Gender differences in weight-related attitudes and behaviors among overweight and obese adults in the United States. *American Journal of Men's Health,* January 15.

CHAPTER 9: FOOLPROOF THE CLEANSE: SIMPLE SECRETS THAT MAKE IT EASY

Aljuraiban, G.S., et al. The impact of eating frequency and time of intake on nutrient quality and Body Mass Index: the INTERMAP Study, a Population-Based Study. *Journal of the Academy of Nutrition and Dietetics* 115: 528–536.

Kong, A., et al. 2012. Self-monitoring and eating-related behaviors are associated with 12-month weight loss in postmenopausal overweight-to-obese women. *Journal of the Academy of Nutrition and Dietetics* 112: 1428–1435.

Watanabe, Y., et al. 2014. Skipping breakfast is correlated with obesity. *Journal of Rural Medicine* 9: 51–58.

CHAPTER 11: AFTER-TOX MEAL PLANS

Abdull Razis, A.F., and Noor, N.M. 2012. Cruciferous vegetables: dietary phytochemicals for cancer prevention. *Asian Pacific Journal of Cancer Prevention* 14: 1565–1570.

Chen, L., et al. 2014. Phytochemical properties and antioxidant capacities of various colored berries. *Journal of the Science of Food and Agriculture* 94: 1800–1888.

Dreher, M.L., and Davenport, A.J. 2013. Hass avocado composition and potential health effects. *Critical Reviews in Food Science and Nutrition* 53: 738–750.

Huang, W.I., et al. 2013. Bioactive natural constituents from food sources—potential use in hypertension prevention and treatment. *Critical Reviews in Food Science and Nutrition* 53: 615–630.

Liu, R.H., 2013. Health-promoting components of fruits and vegetables in the diet. *Advances in Nutrition* 4: 384S–392S.

Story, E.N., et al. 2010. An update on the health effects of tomato lycopene. *Annual Review of Food Science and Technology* 1:189–210.

CHAPTER 12: DETOX YOUR LIFESTYLE

Kraft, T.L., and Pressman, S.D. 2012. Grin and bear it: the influence of manipulated facial expression on the stress response. *Psychological Science* 23: 1372–1378.

O'Leary, K., and Dockray, S. 2015. The effects of two novel gratitude and mindfulness interventions on well-being. *Journal of Alternative and Complementary Medicine* 21: 243–245.

Wheatley, D. 2005. Medicinal plants for insomnia: a review of their pharmacology, efficacy and tolerability. *Journal of Psychopharmacology* 19: 414–421.

INDEX

Page numbers in **boldface** refer to recipes.

bell peppers, 44, 206
 Roasted Red Pepper,
  153
berries, 26, 49, 51–52, 96,
  178, 191, 192
 Berries with Brazil
  Nuts, **130**
 Triple-layer Berry
  Cheesecake, **249–50**
 Very Berry Smoothie,
  237
 *see also specific
  berries*
beta-carotene, 25, 44,
  45, 94
binge response, 14, 15,
  19, 100, 174, 178,
  226–27
black beans, 36, 207
 Black Bean Burgers
  with Slaw, **157**
blackberries, 51, 186
black pepper, 55
Bliss Balls, **247–48**
bloat, bloating, 7, 12, 15,
  48, 55, 60, 61, 63,
  94, 106, 108, 177, 189,
  193, 212–13, 215
 bowel movements
  and, 23, 106
 cooked foods and, 94
 dairy products and,
  64, 109, 195
 detox and, 5, 82,
  89, 98
 fiber and, 100
 natural diuretics and,
  45, 51
 potassium and, 192
 raw-food detoxes and,
  16–17
 from salt, 65, 106, 215
 from sugar, 67, 215
blood sugar levels, 49,
  53, 56, 95, 194, 215,
  225
 carbs and, 35
 cooked vs. raw
  vegetables and, 94
 fiber and, 23–25
 juicing and, 12, 118
 and plant-based
  diet, 22
 skipping meals and,
  167
 sleep loss and, 224
 snacking and, 91, 167
blueberries, 49, 51, 186,
  191, 206

body:
 after-tox maintenance
  of, *see* Sharp
  Lifetime Diet
 before and after
  photos of, 81–82
 cleansing of, *see*
  5-Day Detox
 deep breathing and,
  177
 exercise and, *see*
  exercise
 free radicals and,
  25, 48
 natural detoxification
  by, 6–7, 26, 111
 pH balance and,
  30–32, 109
 self-image and
  awareness of, 82,
  83–84, 163, 165, 171,
  174, 195
 sleep loss and, 63, 92,
  224
 water essential to
  functioning of, 57
 see also digestion,
  digestive system
body brushing, 174
body fat, 36, 63, 90, 97
 cellulite and, 29–30
 dietary fats and, 197
 hydration and, 57
 in men vs. women,
  103–5
 multiple meals and,
  167
 obesogens and, 27–28
 toxins accumulating in,
  7, 26
 types of, 104–5
bowel movements,
  elimination:
 fiber and, 12, 15, 23, 49,
  106
 raw foods and, 92
 water essential for, 57
 see also colon health;
  constipation;
  diarrhea
brain, brain function:
 alcohol and, 63
 antioxidants and, 19
 appetite and, 23, 49
 blood flow and, 171
 juice fasts and, 13
 oils, fats and, 19, 49,
  197
 omega-3s and, 202

brazil nuts, 40
 Berries with Brazil
  Nuts, **130**
breakfast, 91, 166–67
 detox recipes for,
  122–29
 Eggs-cellent Breakfast,
  129
 post-detox recipes for,
  235–38
breast cancer, 7, 40
broccoli, 19, 26, 27, 43,
  44, 202
bromelain, 192
buckwheat, 194
burgers:
 Black Bean Burgers
  with Slaw, **157**
 fast-food, 20, 213
 Homemade Burgers
  with Caramelized
  Onions, **240–41**

cabbage, purple, 19,
  43, 44
 Cabbage Patch Wraps,
  243–44
 Cleansing Cabbage
  Bowl, **158**
caffeine, 6, 19, 63–64, 66,
  100, 110, 225
 decaffeinating process
  and, 168
 headaches and, 99
 sleep loss and, 225
 in tea, 59–61, 168
calcitriol, 90
calcium, 20, 36, 44, 39,
  66, 109
 absorption of, 90, 94,
  203
 in goat's vs. cow's
  milk, 196
 in hemp milk, 196
 sleep and, 225
 in soy, 42, 43
 supplements, 202
 and vitamin D, 203
cancer, 36, 44, 45, 46,
  49, 51, 52, 56, 60, 67,
  184, 193
 acidic diet and, 108
 antioxidants and, 27,
  48, 168
 free radicals and,
  25–26
 household chemicals
  and, 220
 and obesity, 107

nutrients, nutrition
(*cont.*)
 detox functions of, *see*
 toxic avengers
 in fats and oils, 197–99
 freshness of food and,
 206
 as key component of
 5-Day Detox, 17, 22
 muscle growth and,
 106
 oxidation and, 19
 plant-based, 22–25
 popular detoxes and,
 12–17
 raw foods and, 92, 94
 in superfood powders,
 96–98
 in supplements, 201–4
 toxins, food additives
 and, 63, 66, 75, 217
nuts, 19, 23, 27, 31, 32, 35,
 39–40, 105, 151, 168,
 192, 217
 see also specific nuts

oatmeal, Lean Clean
 Oatmeal, **236**
oats, 53, 168–69
 Energizing Oats, **125**
 Energizing Oats
 (postdetox), **187**
obesity, 12–13, 23
 factors contributing to,
 12–13, 23, 66
 and sexual function,
 107
obesogens, 27–29, 104
 and cellulite, 29
oils, *see* fats and oils
omega-3 fatty acids, 36,
 42, 97, 108, 196, 197,
 198, 202
omega-6 fatty acids,
 198
onions, 27, 45
 Homemade Burgers
 with Caramelized
 Onions, **240–42**
organs, 90, 107, 108, 172,
 197
 natural detoxing by, 7,
 9–10, 17, 19, 106, 174
 skin as, 10
 toxins and, 65
 yoga and, 172
 see also digestion,
 digestive system
osteoporosis, 42, 66, 202

overeating, 99, 171, 174,
 178, 212, 217, 218
 emotional issues and,
 226
 fiber and, 23
 food portioning
 and, 79
 forgiveness and, 179

packaged foods, 65, 71,
 73, 184, 217
pancakes:
 High Protein Pancakes,
 237
 Love Pancakes, **126**
Parkinson's, 7
perchloroethylene, 220
persistent organic
 pollutants (POPs), 7
pesticides, 6, 7, 75, 97,
 133, 184, 214
pH (acid-alkaline)
 balance, 30–32
 see also acidic foods,
 acidity; alkaline
 foods, alkalinity
Phandis, Helen, 71
photography, food,
 205–6
photos, before and after,
 81–82
phytochemicals, 12, 25,
 36, 39, 43, 44, 45,
 46, 49, 51, 52, 108,
 109, 189, 202
 in cooked foods, 94
 decaffeinating process
 and, 168
 detoxifying, 26–28
 in organic vs. inorganic
 foods, 75
 in raw foods, 92
phytoestrogens, 109
Piña Colada Smoothie,
 246–47
pineapple, 192
pizza, Cauliflower Pizza,
 242
plant-based foods, 18,
 22–25, 53, 217
 digestive system
 and, 64
 eating out and, 212
 fiber in, 22–25, 216
 and insulin
 sensitivity, 22
 and muscle mass, 110
 pH balance and, 31–32
PMS, 7

polyunsaturated fats, 197,
 198, 199
POPs (persistent organic
 pollutants), 7
portion size, 34, 43, 79,
 91, 98, 100, 111–13, 119,
 187, 207, 213
potassium, 31, 36, 39, 44,
 45, 48, 49, 51, 52, 92,
 97, 98, 109, 190, 192
probiotics, 196, 203
produce, washing of, 133
protein, 52, 53, 91, 97,
 107, 151, 186, 194, 196,
 202, 207
 animal, 64–65, 69
 best sources of, 192–93
 cleansing, 35–43
 gluten, 168
 High-Protein Pancakes,
 237
 hunger satisfied with,
 35, 111
 in juice, 13
 plant vs. animal, 35,
 109
 serving size for, 192
protein powders and
 shakes, commercial,
 65, 109
pumpkin seeds, 39, 40,
 168
 Apple with Sunflower
 or Pumpkin Seeds,
 130

quinoa, 52–53, 109, 129

radishes, 46
raspberries, 51–52, 107–8
Raw Carrot Cupcakes,
 248–49
Raw Chocolate Mousse
 Tarts, **250**
raw food:
 detoxes, 12, 16–17
 digestion and, 92–94,
 167
 pesticides and, 133
red pepper, Roasted Red
 Pepper, **153**
rice milk, 196
ripening, artificial, 6
Roasted Red Pepper, **153**
rolls, Sushi Rolls, **143–44**

salads:
 Colorful Crunch Salad,
 140

ABOUT THE AUTHOR

NIKKI SHARP is a health and fitness expert who focuses on wellness and living a healthier, cleaner, greener lifestyle. After years of working as an international model, Nikki started to realize that she was tired of always wanting to be "skinny" and started pursuing her new passion: health. Through her work as a health coach and wellness blogger, Nikki's mission is to spread the knowledge of healthy living for the mind, body, and soul. She currently resides in Los Angeles.

nikkisharp.com

facebook.com/nikkisharplimited

@NikkiRSharp

instagram.com/nikkisharp

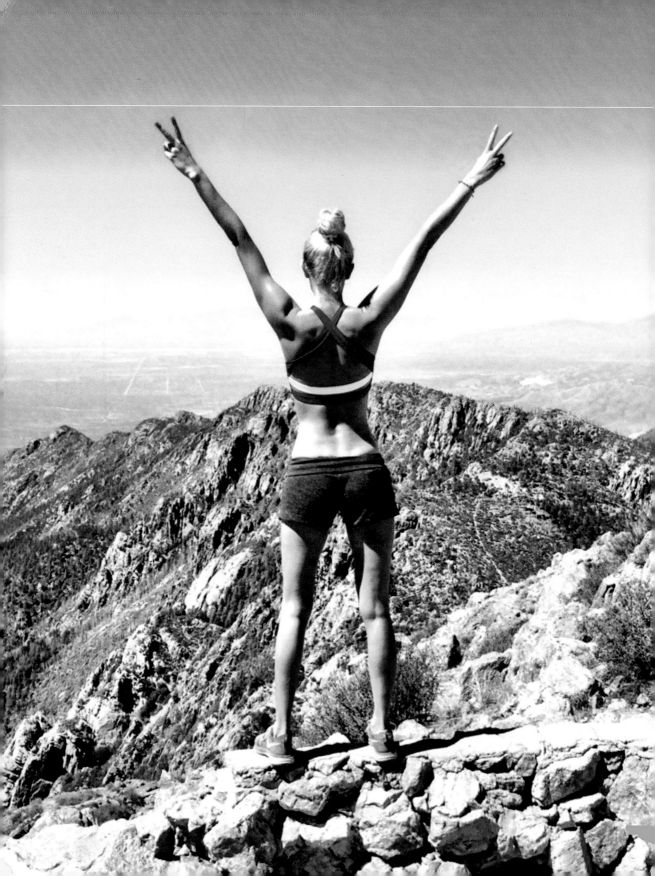